Mentally Create Your Ideal Weight

✦

Use the Power of Your Mind to Change Your Body

Lance Morton

iUniverse, Inc.

New York Lincoln Shanghai

Mentally Create Your Ideal Weight
Use the Power of Your Mind to Change Your Body

iUniverse, Inc.

For information address:
iUniverse, Inc.
2021 Pine Lake Road, Suite 100
Lincoln, NE 68512
www.iuniverse.com

ISBN: 0-595-30405-2

Printed in the United States of America

Mentally Create Your Ideal Weight

I would like to dedicate this book to my sister and our deceased mother.

My mom always believed that I was kind, brilliant, and handsome. Even without one shred of tangible evidence, my mother believed that I was destined to do something important that would help others. I know my mother would have been proud of this book and would have viewed it as a significant work for the betterment of mankind. That was just her way.

My sister supported me and encouraged me when I walked away from a $60,000 a year job, just four years from retirement, to follow my dream and become a hypnotist. She believed in me when no other living person would or even could. Thanks sister; our mother lives in you.

Contents

Introduction

This is a very, simple practical book designed to help you achieve your weight loss goals with no pain and minimum effort. It does not require hard work and painful self-denial to practice the principles presented here. It does require the use of imagination and the exercise of faith.

This book is written for the millions of people who know that they are overweight not because of a rare medical condition, but rather due to their behaviors or habits.

None of the core ideas in this book are originally mine. My only claim to originality is the way that I explain concepts, which were taught to me in clinical terms. I freely admit that my explanations often err on the side of oversimplification.

My belief is that you do not want to be able to lecture on brain theory; you just want to lose weight easily and enjoyably, and you want that weight loss to be permanent. That is what this book is about. These principles have worked for me and countless others and they will work for you. So read, think, and become thin.

1

The Reason Why This Time Will Be Different

My guess is that this is not the first time that you have read a book on weight loss. My guess is this is not the first weight loss program in which you have invested. I am even going to go out on a limb and guess that you already know a great deal about weight loss. I am also going to guess that none of your past efforts to become thin and stay thin have worked as well as you would have liked. I know your efforts are genuine, and you deserve to have the success that you have tried so hard to obtain.

I know as well as you do about the pain of being overweight. It powerfully and negatively impacts every area of your life. According to statistics compiled by Weight Loss International, 65 percent of Americans are losing the battle with weight management, and 31 percent are obese (compared to 23 percent in 1994). The truth is, most Americans are valiantly fighting to lose weight. One of the main reasons we are losing this battle is that a very accurate, powerful, and little understood science is being used against us.

Here is a direct quote from Weight Loss International: "Lifestyles have become hectic, and maintaining a proper body weight sadly has been swamped by *the marked increase in the consumption of fast foods*."

The science of suggestion is being used to make us fat and to keep us that way. At the risk of sounding like a comic book hero, my goal is to help you use this power of suggestion for good instead of evil.

You are no stranger to the science of suggestion. You come in contact with it and are influenced by it at least one hundred times a day. The science of suggestion has many names. Here are a few: advertising, sales, marketing, teaching methodology, and hypnosis.

Now don't get me wrong: advertisers and marketers are not vicious, evil people. They are among some of the most creative people in society. They don't especially want us to be fat and miserable; they just want to make money. They have learned to use the science of suggestion to convince us to eat cheaply made foods that are high in carbohydrates and low in protein. They have convinced us to prefer these types of food and to consume them in mass quantities. The more we eat, the more money they make, and the fatter we get. The fatter we get, the more we *can* eat.

Just as a magician cannot allow the audience to understand how he performs his illusions, advertisers don't want you to know the tricks of their trade. *In this book, I will reveal to you their secrets as they apply to weight loss.* You will not only learn to defend yourself from this subtle technology, but you will learn to use the power of suggestion to create for yourself the body that you desire and deserve.

The first step is to recognize when your suggestibility is influenced in a way that doesn't support your weight loss goal. To illustrate this point, let me give you an example of a typical television commercial that manipulates your suggestibility to behave in ways that will make you fat.

The scene opens. Jerry Jones, the owner of the Dallas Cowboys, is sitting in what looks to be a luxurious penthouse suite. He is talking to Deon Sanders, who at the time was generally considered to be the best defensive halfback in football. Deon played *both* professions; football and professional baseball. It was well known that he had just agreed to play for the Dallas Cowboys for the sum of $35 million dollars.

The dialogue starts with Jones saying: "Deon, what will it take to make you a Dallas Cowboy? Fifteen or 20 million dollars?" Deon just smiles and says, "Both." Jones looks chagrinned, and the commercial cuts away to a pizza advertisement. The announcer asks, "What do you want? One pizza or both?" The answer is obviously both because we want to be like Deon.

In this typical example, the advertisers manipulate our suggestibility by sending mixed associations. Obviously, it is better to have $35 million dollars than it is to have either $15 or $20 million, but if you are trying to lose weight, is it really better to eat one pizza or both pizzas?

The message creates positive associations in our mind: the dream of riches and fame, the opportunity to be like one of our favorite athletes, and the chagrin of an unpopular owner. The obvious humor of the commercial associates pleasure in our unconscious mind and creates suggestibility to go get two pizzas instead of one.

The bottom line is that such manipulation of our suggestibility works. If it didn't, the pizza chain would not spend millions of dollars to run the commercial. The commercial is written, directed, and produced to appeal to our uncon-scious mind *using known principles of human suggestibility.*

The science of suggestion could have just as easily been used to create an entirely different suggestibility in the reader. Imagine this commercial, if you will. The scene opens with Deon Sanders in the doctor's office, and the doctor tells him that he has turf toe. Deon looks anxious and asks if the doctor can fix it. The doctor says, "No, but I can induce turf toe in the other foot so *both* feet will match." The doctor laughs maniacally and says, "So what's it gonna be, Deon, one toe or *both?*" Now Deon looks chagrinned.

The commercial could then cut away to a scene where the slender, athletic, well-built Deon with his *one* toe bandaged is eating *one* pizza. At the table next to him, a fat, unattractive, unknown guy could be choking down two pizzas and holding his belly in obvious pain. The message here would be obvious: one pizza is better than two pizzas.

The truth is, if you watch television, you will see countless commercials that create the same type of suggestibility as displayed in the commercial that actually ran, and you will never see a commercial like the one that I've described.

Let's face it: Americans are bombarded by advertisements that alter our sug-gestibility in ways that cause us to be fat and physically unfit. The good news is, once we recognize what they are doing, we can defend ourselves from this manip-ulation. The better news is that once we understand the simple principles of the science of suggestion, we can use this science to create the type of thoughts that will allow us to become thin and stay thin.

Simply by reading this book and practicing the exercises presented here, you will be able to master the simple principles of the science of suggestion so that you can become thin and stay thin.

2

Why Me

I intend for this book to influence millions of people *to discover their own ability to become thin, enjoying life more than ever before.* Who am I to write a book of such importance? Why should you believe that the suggestions in this book can and will work for you? What are my qualifications? These are good questions.

Honestly, my inspiration came from frustration, desperation, and finally perspiration. Not unlike many other people, I spent 20 years of my life engaged in an occupation for which I had no passion, little interest, and not much aptitude.

I taught history, psychology, and sociology at the high school level for five years. I loved teaching, and I had an aptitude for it. However, I wanted more money than I could make as a teacher so I earned a M.Ed. and became a school principal in the Texas Public Schools Systems. I was employed as a principal for 20 years. Even though I admire and respect the work of public school principals, it was not work that I ever really wanted to do or for which I was well suited. I spent 20 years of my life feeling like the proverbial one-arm paperhanger.

I didn't want to punish people; I wanted to encourage them. I didn't want to exert external control over people; I wanted to influence their hearts and minds. I didn't want to force people to comply with rules; I wanted to challenge them to look at their problems in new and different ways.

However, I got caught up in trying to make a living to support my family. I enjoyed learning about teaching methodology, and my 20 years as a principal allowed me to learn effective teaching from literally hundreds of outstanding teachers. I never did an observation without learning some distinction with regard to teaching.

I loved the teaching aspect of my job, but the many details and management issues were mind numbing to me. I had a need for mental stimulation that went beyond what was available in my job as principal. Over the 20 years, I read extensively about human motivation, brain theory, philosophy, theology, sales, marketing, psychology, success literature, meta-physics, and hypnosis.

I literally read hundreds of books. I earned my first hypnosis certification from the Hypnosis Motivation Institute in 1996, and I earned another certification from American Institute of Hypnotherapy in 2001.

From my readings and my studies, I began to discover that there exists a group of core principles that remained the same whether I was reading about teaching methodology, psychology, marketing, success literature, philosophy, meta-physics, or hypnosis. Each discipline explained the concepts differently but *essentially they were the same concepts! They are universal truths!*

The books contained truths. I discovered that by understanding one discipline, I was able to recognize the same concept presented in a different way. My understanding of these concepts was mostly intellectual. I was not applying these principles to my life. More importantly, I was not practicing these principles in my life.

My life was not working for me. My marriage of 19 years failed, and I found myself living alone in a strange town separated from children, friends, and the woman for whom I cared. I had allowed my life to degenerate to the point that I began to daydream about the fact that I had purchased a large life insurance policy. If anything happened to me; my children would be taken care of financially.

For me it was a time of desperate isolation and bitter loneliness. I felt like a complete failure, and I began to question whether or not I had ever done anything truly worthwhile to help people. It was then I began to realize that almost all my thoughts were about me. One truth I knew from all my reading was *if you wish to be truly happy, you must do something for someone else.*

My mother had instilled in me the belief that I was destined to do something to help others. I quit focusing on what was wrong with my life. *I begin to focus on what I could do to help others. The universe seemed to shout the answer to me. In my soundless solitude, I begin to listen!*

I ate lunch in the teacher's lounge and heard teachers talking about how fat and miserable they were. They talked of how disgusted they were by their own bodies in the mirror. They talked about how bad and unhealthy they felt and looked. Someone said that they were so fat they had lost their sex drive. Someone said, "Forget sex, I would just like to be able to climb a flight of stairs." Someone else mentioned how much her joints ached because of her excess pounds. A lady cried as she talked about an overweight friend dying of a heart attack at an early age.

I went to my office where I had to discipline some children for making fun of an overweight classmate. It seemed everywhere I looked people suffered from being overweight. The collective pain people felt from being overweight was overwhelming. At the time, I was uncomfortable and struggling to keep my stomach sucked in so that I would not pop the last button on my paints. It is often during quiet moments such as this when man has an epiphany. As my button blew, I had my epiphany.

I began to use my hypnosis training, working part-time to help people lose weight. When I wasn't working with clients, I was contemplating how to integrate all that I had learned over the course of a lifetime into one simple workable system that enabled people to lose weight successfully and *enjoy the process*.

My clients began to get good results, and I discovered my mission in life. I began to systematically distill all the knowledge from the master teachers whose words had influenced me and to make that knowledge relevant to one topic and one topic only. That topic was weight loss.

I condensed and simplified what my teachers had taught me about life, making those principles specifically relevant to weight loss. Often I would study, contemplate, and write for 10 hours at a time. During a four-month period, I rarely slept for over four hours a night.

During this time, I developed a burning desire to help people end their suffering from being overweight. I became so passionately committed to this proposition that I quit my job. I just walked away from the only profession I had known for the last 20 years. I left a $60,000 a year job just four years short of retirement to build a business that almost no one believed would support my family.

I moved back near my children and opened the "Hypnosis Weight Loss Center." As I worked with and listened to my clients, I began to learn simple ways to explain the concepts that I had been learning over the last 20 years. I successfully used the principles that I had discovered in my own life to lose 40 pounds of fat while gaining 10 pounds of muscle.

I had no idea from where my next dollar was coming or how I would get clients. I operated with a "Field of Dreams" mentality. "Build it, and they will come!" All I had was a burning white-hot desire to help people change their lives by changing their thoughts and their bodies. It was then that I developed faith, imagination, and persistence.

Amazingly, clients began to come to me. Many of my clients became successful, and I became euphoric. I had found my mission in life. I knew my mission was to teach people to become thin and stay thin in the most simple, practical, and enjoyable way possible.

Who am I? I'm just an average guy who discovered his mission late in life. I am honored that you are reading this book, and I will be delighted–but not surprised–when I learn that you became thin and stayed thin.

3

It All Starts With a Thought

Look around you. Everything in material reality once started as a thought in someone's mind. All music, literature, art, and architecture started as a thought in someone's mind. The cars you see, the furniture you sit on, the computer you use, and the cell phone you talk on all started as a thought in someone's mind.

This principle is true with regard to weight loss. Barring disease, famine, or abject poverty, before you can lose weight you must have the thought of losing weight. Since you are reading this book, I am quite certain that you have already met this first prerequisite to weight loss.

I believe that the greatest gift and power that we possess as human beings is our *ability to control our own thoughts*. At this moment you can choose to think of something pleasant or something sad. You can choose to think about eating, or working, or having sex, or any of a vast number of other thoughts. In each and every moment of your life, the choice is always yours regardless of the circumstances surrounding you.

If you are overweight right now, it is because you choose to think about eating and exercise in ways that cause you to be overweight. This book will teach how to think about eating and exercise in ways that will empower you to reach your ideal weight and size.

Think about it! Before you eat anything, you *think* about eating. There is no other way to accomplish the act of eating. Because we have the ability to choose our thoughts, we have the ability to control our eating. By reading this book, you will learn many simple, painless techniques to recondition your thoughts about eating. Eventually, you will train your thoughts to become as *automatic as your breathing*, thus ending the struggle with your weight forever.

When you change the way you think about eating, your behaviors will change. Then your weight will have to change; it will simply have no other choice.

I am not into conspiracy theories, but the truth is, the media doesn't want you to know this fact: *you can become your ideal weight and size without the use of drugs, herbs, diets, or strenuous exercise.* In this country, billions of dollars are spent on advertising campaigns designed to convince you to think in ways that lead you to overeat.

Advertisers are willing to spend millions of dollars for 30 seconds of airtime because they know that in those 30 seconds, via hypnosis technology, they can create suggestibility for you to eat cheaply-made, high carbohydrate foods with little nutritional value. They know they can convince a percentage of their viewers to *want* to eat this type of food in large quantities.

The media is very good at creating images and associations in your imagination that convince you that it is highly desirable to eat fattening foods. These advertisements don't mention that eating these foods will cause you to be overweight, sap you of energy, and destroy your sex life. They don't tell you that being overweight significantly increases a person's risk of life-threatening diseases such as diabetes, heart disease, stroke, high blood pressure, and some types of cancer. Americans are being bombarded with suggestions for eating foods that are essentially ruinous to your health, happiness, and enjoyment of life. If you eat massive amounts of these foods, the profit margin is even greater for advertisers and retailers.

The truth is, you can defend yourself from these suggestions that are not in your best interest. *You can control your thoughts.* There exists a body of scientific principles that, when followed, will allow you to control your thoughts. It is simply a matter of learning the principles presented in this book and applying them to your life.

If it is really this simple, just a matter of changing how you think, why doesn't everyone do it? I believe everyone doesn't do it because not everyone has the recipe. Think of this book as a recipe book for changing how you think about eating and exercise. The first ingredient in this book is desire, which is the subject of the next chapter.

4

Desire

As humans, we experience lots of different kinds of thoughts. There are musings, wondering thoughts, curious thoughts, humorous thoughts, angry thoughts, and fearful thoughts, etc., but among the types of thoughts, desire is one of the strongest.

Desire is the starting point of all human achievement. Anyone who has ever achieved something very important or difficult has been able to do so because her wish had grown into a desire. As you begin to *learn* to control your thoughts, you will become aware of a great many types of thoughts that leap into your mind unbidden. There are thoughts that can distract, misdirect, and frighten you from achieving your goals. In order to conquer these destructive thoughts, you will have to learn how to harness the power of desire.

You cannot simply hope that you will lose weight or wish that you could be able to lose weight. Those types of thoughts are too weak to help you to achieve your goals. It is not enough to think, "Gee, I would kinda like to lose a few pounds." The simple truth is, if you want to lose weight, you are going to have to develop a burning desire to do so.

A person can choose to develop desire in much the same way that you can choose to develop your physical muscles: through exercise. I am going to give you a simple set of exercises that, when done as instructed, will build your desire to lose weight into a vibrant and powerful force that can and will sweep away weaker thoughts.

Desires are dreams turned into realities just waiting to be born. A desire is so vivid and compelling that you absolutely know that it must come to pass. In order to increase the intensity of a desire, visualize or imagine yourself *already* in possession of the object of your desire. In your imagination, visualize all the pleasure that you will experience when that desire is achieved. See yourself already enjoying your ideal body!

Keep that desire in the forefront of your thoughts. Whatever you pay attention to will grow stronger in your life. Frequently remind yourself that you are in the process of becoming your ideal weight and size. See this desire to become slender as bigger and more powerful than your wish to eat fattening foods. Only associate the word "desire" with your *definite major purpose* of losing weight. Thoughts that run counter to your weight loss goals should never be considered anything more than passing thoughts that will quickly pass and die from lack of attention.

If you have a *passing thought* to eat something that you know is not good for you, picture that thought as a small flame on a tiny candle flickering in the wind. See your desire as a brightly blazing fire with lots of hot, blue coals casting a brilliant light inside a warm and friendly fireplace.

Now watch as a gust of wind blows out the small flame on the candle of the *passing* thought of eating something that is wrong for you. You can watch that tiny flame go out: the smoke lingers for a while and is gone, and as the smoke dissipates into the atmosphere so does the passing thought. Now watch the wind gust into that blazing fire of your desire to lose weight, and watch the fire burn and blaze with more intensity. The wind cannot blow out the fire of true desire. It can only fan it to blaze more brightly than before.

Visit this fire of your desire to lose weight frequently. Exercise your right to chop wood and to place large logs on the hot blue coals of your fire. Feel the comforting warmth of your healthy desire to lose weight. Allow yourself to be warmed and relaxed by the fire of your desire.

By attending to this fire with diligence, you will have done more to insure that you will absolutely become slender than if you had memorized every diet concept on the market. Most overweight people are experts on what they should or shouldn't eat. Just knowing what to do is not enough to insure your weight loss success. The difference between success and failure is directly related to the intensity of the desire to lose weight. You can control your thoughts, and you can control the intensity of those thoughts. *A thought at the highest level of intensity is a desire.*

If you do nothing more than intensify your desire to lose weight to a level of hot white heat, you will absolutely achieve your goal. A desire this strong will find a way to accomplish its mission. It cannot and will not be sidetracked, delayed, or denied.

Discover yourself daydreaming about this fire of your desire and learn to close your eyes and see the flames in brilliant hues of white, blue, yellow, and red as they blaze across the movie screen of your mind's eye.

Practice this imagery whenever you have a moment, or whenever you have a passing thought that doesn't support your weight loss goal. Soon you will find that all those thoughts of eating something bad for you are only weak candles barely flickering in the wind. Simply allow them to be extinguished by your *practiced inattention.* The conscious mind cannot hold two separate thoughts at one time. So if you focus on and concentrate on the brightly blazing fire, all the flickering candles will simply become extinguished.

With practice, you will become good at this imagery. You can find that this inner thought game is very enjoyable and stimulating. You are learning to master your own thoughts, and a person who can master his thoughts can achieve his objectives. Remember: *repetition is the mother of all learning, so keep practicing!*

To further intensify your desire, answer the following questions and write the answers on paper. Answer as completely and with as much specificity as possible. Evoke an emotional response with your writing. When you write something that brings a tear to your eye, underline that portion; the more emotion that you can evoke, the better. Learn to feel this desire as a powerful warming fire burning your excess weight and transforming your fat and cellulite into smoke that lingers for a brief moment and then quickly dissipates into the atmosphere.

- Why do I absolutely *have* to lose weight now?

- If you have been gaining 10 pounds a year, ask yourself what your life will be like 10 years from now when you are 100 pounds more overweight than you are today?

- Think about carrying a 100-pound backpack around for the next 20 years.

- How tired are you?

- How do your muscles feel?

- How do your joints feel?

- What activities do you miss out on?

- How do you move?

- How do you look?

- What is your sex life like?

Continue to ask yourself these types of questions until you can evoke an emotional response. Continue to imagine this bad scenario until it becomes obvious that you *cannot* allow this to happen.

Find a place to be alone and ask yourself loudly, with passion, "Is this the kind of life I am willing to accept or am I better than this?" Answer in a strong, clear voice that you are better than this and you will not allow this to happen.

Now imagine yourself your ideal weight and size.

- How do you feel?

- How do you look?

- How much more energy do you have?

- How much more fun do you have?

- How much more successful are you?

- What is your sex life like now?

Give yourself some time to answer these questions. When you have finished answering these questions, do the following four steps.

First: Fix in your mind the exact amount that you want to weigh, and put a definite date to it. If you want to lose 50 pounds, allow for a two-pound a week weight loss for the next 25 weeks. Look it up on the calendar, and write the exact date down. Convince yourself that the weight must absolutely be gone by *that date*. Make yourself a solemn promise to lose the weight by *that date*. Tell yourself that you will keep your promises to yourself, no matter what.

Second: Determine exactly what you intend to give in return for becoming your ideal weight and size. For example, write: "I will read this book and enthusiastically engage in all the activities presented until I achieve my goal of becoming my ideal weight and size. I will continue to read this book and practice the techniques presented here *until* I become my ideal weight and size, even if I have to read this book over and over!"

Third: Begin to develop a plan to lose all the weight that you desire. In chapter seven, I will teach you how to do this step-by-step. For now, your chief concern is to read this book in its entirety.

Fourth: Read the following statement out loud twice daily: once just before retiring at night and once after arising in the morning. As you read, see and feel yourself already at your ideal weight and size, read this statement with passion and confidence:

"I will achieve my desire of becoming my ideal weight and size by intensifying that desire. I will keep this burning desire to be healthier, leaner, fitter, and more attractive in the forefront of my thoughts. I will imagine myself at my ideal weight and size and I will experience in my imagination all the pleasure that achieving my goal will bring. My blazing desire enables me to easily learn and practice the techniques presented in this book. My desire to become slender grows stronger with each and every passing day."

Following these four steps does not require hard work, but it does require an open mind, the use of your imagination, and persistence—and one other thing: faith! Faith is the subject of the next chapter.

5

Faith

In order to achieve your weight loss goal, you will have to have faith that *you can* achieve your goals. Faith is that very powerful emotion that gives you staying power to pursue your goals, especially when it doesn't seem like your weight loss program is working.

The kind of weight loss that we are talking about is not instantaneous. You don't begin to practice your mental exercises one day, master them the next, and lose all the weight you desire on the third day. It will take about 28-33 days to master the principles taught in this program. Once learned, this new way of thinking will become an *automatic* part of your thought process.

When this program begins to work, you will *not* notice changes in your weight. First you will notice that your *thoughts* begin to change. Not all of your thoughts will change, but *some thoughts will begin to change.* When you notice that a thought is changing, then your faith will begin to grow. When you pay attention to your own thinking process, you are essentially applying fertilizer to the thought that you desire to grow.

Next you will notice that your behaviors are changing. Look for signs of your changing behavior. These signs that your behavior is in fact changing will nurture and develop your faith. Realize that as your behaviors change, sooner or later, your body will have to change.

Next you will notice that your clothes are looser, you move easier, and you are losing weight. Realize that if you are capable of losing even one pound by chang-ing your thoughts about eating and exercise, then you are capable of losing two pounds, three pounds, etc.

Notice all your positive changes in thought, behavior, and weight loss. *Noth-ing builds the faith muscle like success.* Acknowledge your successes as proof posi-tive that you will absolutely reach your goal.

Don't let temporary setbacks diminish your faith. Remember that no one can achieve success without having setbacks. "Every failure brings with it the seeds of an equivalent success." Allow the winds of failure to fan the fire of your desire.

In this book, you will learn how to condition yourself for success through your failures. You will be able to begin looking at your failures as opportunities to recondition your automatic thinking so that your positive conditioning will be even stronger than before. In this way, temporary defeat can be used to build your faith.

You can begin to build your faith by increasing your self-confidence. First you should know that *you have the ability to achieve your weight loss goals.* I have done it, and so have countless others, and so can you. If you ever doubt that you can achieve your goals, simply *pretend* that you can. Never speak a doubt out loud. Counter every doubtful thought with an "I can" thought, even if you have to pretend. The power of pretend is so important that I have dedicated an entire chapter to it.

If you do not know what to do in any moment, you can always improve the situation by having a positive thought replace a negative one. Then quickly act upon the positive thought. The action can be small and simple, but the timing is crucial. By acting quickly on your positive thoughts, you create positive momentum. Promise yourself that you will take persistent and continuous action toward achieving your goal. Practice being aware of and guiding your thoughts.

Know that the dominating thoughts of your mind eventually reproduce themselves in your actions, behaviors, and outward physical appearance. In quiet moments, concentrate your thoughts on how you will look when you are your ideal weight and size.

Throughout the day, imagine yourself lean. Learn to daydream about being fit, firm, healthy, and attractive. Know that you are doing more than daydreaming. You are in fact creating the body of your dreams in your mind. *Remember all creation first begins in the mind.*

Your faith can be built through the use of affirmations, self-hypnosis, autosuggestions, the power of questions, and the power of pretend. There will be more discussion of these techniques later in the book. All the techniques mentioned absolutely work, and all employ the active use of your imagination. Imagination is the subject of the next chapter.

6

Imagination

All dreams come from our imaginations. *Desire is given shape and form through the active use of imagination.* It is possible for your imagination to become weak from lack of use, and it is possible to build the power of your imagination through active daily use.

Imagination is the key to losing all the weight that you desire. Time and time again throughout this book, you will be asked to use your imagination. Children instinctively know the pleasure of allowing their imaginations to run wild. If you have ever played with an imaginary friend, fought a dragon and rescued a princess, become an astronaut, or a cowboy, or a secret agent, or a beauty queen, or played mom and dad; you know how enjoyable and exciting the use of the imagination can be.

Adults are taught to put away things of the imagination and focus on reality, but the truth is, *all reality begins in the imagination!* There is simply no other place to begin the work of creative genius. If it doesn't happen in the imagination first, it just doesn't happen.

Your imagination is automatic. You really do not have a choice of using it or not. Your imagination is irrepressible. You will always imagine something. The question is: Will you imagine something that empowers you to accomplish your dreams and goals, or will you use your imagination to bring the thing you fear into existence?

How is thinking of yourself as an unhealthy, fat, unattractive, lethargic person more real than thinking of yourself as a healthy, fit, firm, lean, energetic, attractive, poised, and self-confident person? It requires the same amount of energy or effort in the imagination to think a positive thought as it does to think a negative one. It is true many people will gladly share and reinforce your own negative thoughts about your ability to lose weight, and yet this reinforcement of your negative thought does not decrease the energy used to think the thought.

How many times have you heard someone say, "After you get to be 40 years old, something happens to the body and you can't lose weight anymore?" We might nod our heads complacently in agreement and mumble something about how we are not as young as we used to be. We might as well throw in the statement that we are not as short as we were when we were born. Though the statements heretofore mentioned are undeniably true, they do not empower us to achieve our desires. It is therefore essentially a waste of mental energy. That same mental energy *could be* channeled to give life to our positive thoughts.

The suggestion that people over 40 are automatically going to gain weight is obviously erroneous. One does not have to look far to see many examples of people that are leaner, fitter, and healthier in their 40s than they were in their 30s. When I was 38, I was soft, out of shape, and I weighed 208 pounds. At the time of this writing, I am 48 years old. I now weigh 185 pounds, and I am a leaner, fitter, and healthier then I was ten years ago. The majority of my improvement came during a five-month period when I began to rediscover the power of my imagination. I learned to use my imagination to develop the physique that I desired.

The principles I used are the exact same ones that you will learn by reading this book. All the principles presented in this book require the use of your active imagination. When they are applied as I suggest–*they will work!* It will require no more effort for you to use you imagination in a positive way than it does for you to use it negatively. If you are overweight now, it is because you have allowed your imagination to think about eating and exercising in ways that cause you to be overweight.

Do not be concerned if other people do not share your knowledge that you will become your ideal weight and size. When Marconi had the inspiration to invent radio and wireless communication and he tried to verbalize the concept to his friends, they had him committed to a psychiatric hospital for observation. However, his desire was so strong and his imagination so vivid that he transformed the concept of radio and wireless communication into reality for billions of people. Think about it: if Marconi could harness the power of his imagination in the face of the ridicule of his friends, it should not be "mission impossible" for you to use your imagination to gain the body you desire and deserve.

To assist in the development of your imagination, find yourself a picture of someone who has the body that you want, and imagine your face on that body. Hang pictures of that person in your bedroom and bathroom, and imagine yourself with his or her body. Find an actor or actress who has a body that you would like to have and rent their movies. Identify with their characters, and see yourself using your body to perform like they do.

Emulation of another person can fire the imagination. Keep in mind that they are just people like yourself that have no doubt learned to think about eating and exercise in similar ways to what you are learning in this book. Almost every performer has fired up his or her imagination by having a fellow performer that they strive to be like. Never underestimate the power of having a good role model.

Think about what you would do if you had your ideal body, and then do it in your imagination. Remember everything that actually happens begins in the imagination. Spend a few minutes each day imagining a pleasurable way in which you will be able to use your ideal body.

Remember: all dreams start in the imagination. No power on earth is greater than your imagination. *When you have learned to control and use the pure dynamic power of your imagination in conjunction with the other principles and techniques presented here, you will be your ideal weight and size.*

Through the active use of your imagination, you will be able to change your habits. Once you have firmly established new habits, *the struggle* with weight management will be over.

7

The Seven Highly Effective Habits of Thin People

Stephen Covey wrote a book that I believe is a modern day classic. The book was called the *"Seven Habits of Highly Effective People."* When I began my Hypnosis Weight Loss Practice, I could not help but notice that I had discovered seven habits of thin people. If you master the seven habits presented in this chapter, you will absolutely *think yourself thin for life!*

My philosophy in doing hypnosis weight loss with my clients is to make minimal changes that will result in maximum weight loss over time. The seven habits contained in this chapter don't require you to make drastic or painful changes in your lifestyle. Once again, you are simply asked to understand the concepts presented and to practice persistently the principles until they become habits.

I have included the desired habit, the problem that requires the habit, and a suggestion for changing the habit. The suggestions listed here should be used both as affirmations and as a self-hypnosis script.

In this book, I will teach you step-by-step how to create this script for yourself, or if you prefer you can simply order my compact disc. On the compact disc, I have already done this for you. Ordering instructions can be found in the back of the book. Even if you decide to order the disk, it is very important to read and understand this chapter, as it will be the practical means by which you achieve your weight loss goal.

The way I have designed this book is to give you the information that you need to begin losing weight right now, today! Later in the book, I will explain why these techniques work, but right now I am giving you *the how* to accomplish your goals and to begin today. Today you *can* begin thinking differently about the foods you eat.

Habit 1. Eat Slowly and Enjoy Your Food

The analogy I use with my patients is this: "I am not suggesting that we do this, but I think it is physically possible for you and I to drink 10 tequila shots in the next 10 minutes. I don't know about you, but 30 minutes later I would be in a lot of trouble. However, if I drank one tequila shot every 15 minutes, I would probably be unable or willing to drink more than five or six shots. To put it another way, simply by slowing down the rate at which I drink, I would be able to drink only 50 to 60 percent of what I could drink by drinking fast."

We eat food so quickly that we do not give our body, or more specifically our unconscious mind, enough time to realize when our stomach is full, comfortable, and satisfied. The unconscious mind has a wisdom that knows when you have eaten just the right amount. Given time, it can be trained to give you a signal that you no longer have a desire to eat past the point of nutritional comfort. The key to this strategy is to *slow down the speed at which you eat.*

Let's do the math for a second. It takes a decrease of about 3,000 calories to lose one pound of bodyweight. If you eat 60 percent of what you have been eating—let's say 3,000 calories a day—you are eating only (3,000 x .60 = 1,800 calories). Now you are eating only 1,800 calories a day, which is 1,200 calories less than you were eating. This means that in five days you will have eaten (5 x 1,200 = 6,000 calories less), which will result in a two-pound weight loss every five days. That will be about 12 pounds per month or 144 pounds per year.

You really can easily and enjoyably obtain this weight loss merely by slowing down the rate at which you eat and consciously enjoying your food more. Think about it: the pleasure of eating is not increased by the speed at which you eat. If this were true, you could eat something that you hated faster and enjoy it more. Let this idea sink into your mind. Think about a hunk of raw liver. If eating fast created enjoyment, you could eat that liver very quickly, and it would taste good. I think that you will agree that this way of thinking makes no sense.

The pleasure of eating is not increased by the amount you eat. If this were true, you could gain pleasure by eating *more* raw liver. It is obvious to our conscious mind that we will not gain more pleasure by eating more raw liver, and yet most us have an unconscious association that says eating more of something is better.

This conditioning is simply not true, because eating too much will lead to feelings of bloating, lethargy, and general bad feelings that may even lead to nausea. When you add these immediate negative consequences of overeating to the many known long-term negative consequences of overeating, it is apparent that eating more brings more pain and less pleasure.

The desire to eat food in large quantities is a predisposition in all animals. One of the most fundamental needs of all animals is to keep from starving to death. Our body has developed the ability to store foods in time of plenty in the form of fat. The purpose of this mechanism is to increase the animal's chances of surviving periods of famine or food shortage.

Animals go through periods in the spring and summer when food is plentiful, and they overeat and become fat. This allows them to survive the fall and winter, a time when foods are not so plentiful. There is a natural fluctuation. The animal surviving the winter will be lean and hard; the same animal will be plump and soft following the summer.

Nature assures that the wild animal does not deviate too far from the norm. Most of us have managed to assure that we have plentiful food supply throughout the year. Failure to reprogram our innate desire to eat all we can we will cause us to be overweight.

Carnivores have a predisposition to eat their food quickly. Historically, all animals including humans, have eaten their food quickly before a bigger and stronger predator could take it away, or before it spoiled. The struggle for survival has deeply imprinted this predisposition into the human brain. It *once served* as a very important survival mechanism. However, today the abundance of food and social inhibitions make it highly unlikely that anyone will take your food from you regardless of how slowly you eat.

At a time when man's average life expectancy was between 20 and 40 years and most people died of starvation, the predisposition to eat all you can as quickly as you can was a very important survival mechanism. However, we live in a society where the average life expectancy is 70-plus years. We live in a society where many more people die from heart failure than starvation. The predisposition to eat all you can as quickly as possible has become a strategy that actually decreases an individual person's life expectancy.

Predispositions that once insured our survival are no longer appropriate in civilized society. Fortunately, we can learn to override this natural tendency to eat too quickly by establishing new associations. If you doubt for a moment that we as humans have the ability to control our genetically encoded predisposition, you should consider that at one time mankind had the drive to discharge excrement whenever and wherever they were. Today, in our society, practically everyone has the ability to control this drive. Controlling the aforementioned behavior is the result of social conditioning. Social conditioning comes from the establishment of new associations or, put more simply, creating new habits. *People have the ability to intentionally create new habits!*

We must begin to think of eating as primarily to insure that our body receives the nutrition that it needs. It is helpful to think of eating as pleasurable as well. *The pleasure of eating comes from enjoying the taste, texture, and aroma of food.* You can better enjoy the taste, texture, and aroma of food when you eat at a more relaxed pace. You can learn to take pleasure in realizing that you are full and satisfied. You can learn to eat less and gain more pleasure.

Suggestion: Whenever I start to eat a meal, I take a deep breath. This breath serves as a reminder to me to eat my food more slowly. I find that I begin to eat my food more and more slowly, savoring each and every bite. I enjoy the taste of my food more and more by eating slowly. I enjoy eating smaller bites, then chewing and swallowing my food before I get another bite. I discover that I am happiest when I eat at a slower pace, and when I do, my food tastes more delicious; I allow my unconscious mind enough time to send a signal to me. When I receive this signal, I know I have eaten just the right amount of food to satisfy my nutritional needs.

I find that when I receive this signal, I am completely nutritionally satisfied. I push my plate six inches from me. As I push my plate from me, I lose my wish to eat any more because I know that each bite past the point of nutritional comfort will only lead to discomfort, a bloating feeling, and a feeling of nausea. In order to avoid these and other unpleasant consequences of overeating, I find that I lose my wish to eat past the point of nutritional comfort. I know when my body is full, and I am happy and content to quit eating when I am full and satisfied.

Habit 2. Preferring to Eat Healthy and Nutritious Foods

It has been my experience from working with clients that most people who are overweight are experts on what they should and shouldn't eat. Time and time again my clients tell me that "I know what kind of foods to eat but I just seem to make bad choices when it comes to eating."

People habitually choose the wrong foods even when they know better. Why? Most people associate a lot of pleasure with eating foods that are fattening and a lot of pain with eating foods that are healthy and nutritious. In chapter 11, I will explain to you how these associations are developed and how we can change them so that you will associate pleasure with eating healthy food and pain with eating food that is fattening. For now, I will give you the suggestions that you need to actually make this change.

Suggestion: Each and every day, I find that I am more drawn to foods that are high in protein and low in carbohydrates. Those foods that promote lean muscle taste better and better with each passing day as I lose the taste for foods that promote the massive accumulation of fatty tissue.

When I eat high protein foods, I can feel my body becoming leaner and more toned; if I try to eat foods that are not good for me, I find that after a bite or two they leave a very unpleasant taste in my mouth. I know that I can cleanse my pallet of this nasty taste by drinking a glass or a bottle of water. Whenever I try to eat foods that are wrong for me, I am reminded that nothing tastes as good as thinness feels.

Habit 3. Eating sweets, snacks, and other fattening foods

Most people associate a lot of pleasure with eating desserts, candy, and fattening foods. In chapter 11, we will look at how these associations are made and why we are able to change these associations to ones that are equally pleasurable but also support our weight loss goal. I am going to give you a suggestion to change this habit so you can begin right now—today—to be in control of your thoughts and to begin to lose all the weight you desire to lose.

Suggestion: Whenever I notice that I have a wish to eat something that is bad for me, I also know that I have a burning desire *to refuse* to eat that very food. I remember that nothing tastes as good as thinness feels. If I still have the wish to eat that fattening food I will *not deny* myself, but I will try to eat that fattening food, one bite at a time. As I try to take the first bite, I will begin to taste all the processed sugar, preservatives, and chemical additives packed into that unhealthy food.

As I chew this food slowly and taste the ingredients, (which are essentially poisonous to my health, happiness, and physical appearance), I will begin to notice that this food leaves a very nasty taste in my mouth. I will find myself losing all desire to eat more than a bite or two. Further, I will find that I can cleanse my pallet of this nasty taste by drinking a glass or a bottle of water.

Note: Never tell yourself that you will not eat something that you *think* you want. Rather, tell yourself that you will eat it if you want it, *but then begin to question whether or not you really want it.* This has to do with a very powerful law of human thinking called the "Law of Reverse Suggestion." This principle is so important that I have dedicated a chapter to its discussion.

Habit 4. Water is the beverage of choice

My ability to help people to get rid of their carbonated drinking habits quickly and easily is what really launched my career as a hypnotist specializing in weight loss. One week after our first session, time and time again my clients returned to me amazed that they had simply lost all desire to drink whatever soft drink to which they formerly thought that they were addicted. It seemed miraculous to them, but it came to be something that I routinely expected to happen.

Once again, let's do a little math to show how big this change can be in your weight loss program. Let us say that you have been drinking four cokes a day at 150 calories per coke (that is 600 calories per day). Remember that it takes about 3,000 calories to lose a pound of weight. So (5 days x 600 calories = 3,000 calories), I admit that math is not my strong suit, but I figure by drinking water instead of cola you will lose one pound every five days, or about six pounds a month, or 72 pounds a year. For some people this is the only modification that they ever need to make to lose all the weight that they desire.

I have found that this change has been produce under hypnosis quickly and easily by the following simple suggestion. (More to come later about why this works.)

Suggestion: Your ability to taste the ingredients in soft drinks is becoming heightened. Whenever you *try* to drink a cola or another soft drink, you will find after a swallow or two that you begin to notice the taste of all the unhealthy artificial flavors and preservatives contained in these highly processed drinks. You can read the ingredients on the can or bottle and begin to taste each ingredient, which is essentially poisonous to your health, happiness, and physical appearance. After a swallow or two, you may notice a very unpleasant and nasty taste in your mouth that serves to increase your thirst. The more you drink, the thirstier you become.

Your lips may become very dry and parched. Your tongue may become thick and acquire a nasty coating, and your throat may become parched and dry, as if you had been in the hot, hot sun of the Sahara desert without water for many days.

The thirst becomes worse with every swallow of cola, but you will find that your thirst is quickly and easily quenched when you drink a glass of water or a bottle of water. As you enjoy the cool and delicious taste of water you will notice that you pallet becomes refreshed; all signs of the nasty-tasting cola have been removed from your mouth.

You feel good about drinking water because you know that it energizes and cleanses your body, and it gives your metabolism a boost as it accelerates your weight loss. You find that cool and delicious water becomes your beverage of choice. You enjoy the clean refreshing taste and find yourself looking forward to drinking water at every opportunity. You enjoy drinking water at meals and in between meals. You know that drinking lots of water is one of the easiest and healthiest things that you can do for yourself.

These suggestions affect you now and become stronger each and every day with each and every breath that you take because you realize that drinking water *is as important as breathing* air, and *drinking lots of water should become as automatic as breathing air.*

Note: I know that the diet drink business is a multi-billion dollar a year industry and I have no desire to incur its displeasure. However I must say that in my experience, I have never run into a single client who claimed they lost weight by changing from a regular soft drink to a diet soft drink.

I have had clients report losing weight by changing from a diet drink to water. Because it is an easy and healthy course of action, I suggest to my clients that diet drinks should be changed to water also. It is beyond my expertise and the scope of this book to debate this subject; I only offer it as a suggestion which has proven helpful to my clients.

Habit 5. Eating the last food of the day prior to 7 P.M.

Humans are essentially biological animals who are influenced by natural cycles. Both research and ancient wisdom have shown us that our metabolism burns the hottest when the sun is at its highest point in the sky. Adjusting for different time zones, this should be somewhere near noon. A more accurate way to determine this for any time of year is to step outside, and see what time it is when the sun is directly overhead.

Once you have established the time, you will know that this is the optimum time to eat your largest meal because your metabolism will burn calories more quickly at this time than at any other. If you wish to make a poor choice in food selection, it would do less damage to do this at noon. Therefore, if it fits with your lifestyle I suggest that you eat your largest meal at noon. Just on the basis of metabolism alone, it would be ideal to eat your last meal between 12 and 2 p.m. **However, I don't suggest that you do this.** The reason I don't suggest this is because it becomes impractical for most people, and it can create a lot of emotional pain. In short, for most people, I think the risk of psychological damage is greater than the potential for metabolic benefit.

Just as noon is the best time to eat for weight loss, the evening and night are the worst times. After 7 p.m. your metabolism slows way down and your body retains more of the calories eaten as fat, which is why I strongly suggest that people eat smaller meals in the evening and that they not eat past 7 p.m. or at least three hours before bedtime.

Suggestion: I find myself wanting to eat my largest meal at noon when the sun is at the highest point in the sky. I am so nutritionally satisfied from my noon meal that I find I a have a growing desire to eat smaller meals in the evening.

I find that I lose the desire to eat past 7 p.m., and when I don't eat past 7 p.m., I find that I fall asleep more quickly and sleep more comfortably. When my head touches the pillow, I drift into a very peaceful slumber, sleeping quickly, deeply, and soundly through the night, dreaming beautiful dreams and waking in the morning refreshed, energized, and highly motivated to follow my weight loss program.

Habit 6. Creating a faster burning metabolism

Sometimes a client will come to me for weight loss and when I ask about their eating habits, they report that they are eating almost nothing. Since eating is largely an unconscious act, many people actually eat much more than they think they do.

Usually, I give them a simple post-hypnotic suggestion to be aware of all they eat during the coming week, and we discover that they have in fact eaten more than they realized. This awareness alone is therapeutic. Once the client is aware of the habits that don't support her weight loss goals, we can precede with the therapy as usual.

Sometimes I discover the client really does not eat very much at all, and they still cannot lose weight. Theoretically, they may not actually be eating enough to support their current weight, and they could be still gaining weight. In every case that I have worked on, when this happens I find that the client has a history of going on starvation diets, losing weight, and then regaining the weight plus some extra pounds. This is the famous yo-yo diet syndrome. When a person has been doing this type of dieting, the unconscious mind becomes convinced that the body is starving to death.

Then the unconscious mind slows all body processes down to convert any available food to fat in order to help the person survive the period of food shortage. In order to do this, the energy level must be low enough so very few calories are burned. The result is a very sluggish metabolism, which converts even the smallest amounts of food into fat.

There are a number of things that a person can do to get their metabolism operating at a normal level again. The first thing I suggest is that the person begin to eat more food. It is important to eat regular meals and to consume a reasonable amount of calories.

As soon as I can get the client's energy level up, I recommend a program of resistance weight training. The increase in lean muscle mass is the most efficient way to turn up the metabolism. Again, I start with simple suggestions to allow the client enjoy the weight training. At first, the suggestion may be to enjoy weight training for at least 20 minutes a day, three times a week, on the days when they are not walking. The objective of the therapy at this point is to attach massive amounts of pleasure to working out and building lean muscle, and massive amounts of pain to failing to work out.

The third thing that I do is hypnotize the client, and at the unconscious level, raise the metabolism. When I first was taught this technique, it seemed a bit airy-fairy to me. I wondered if it was really possible to turn up the metabolism by simply directing the unconscious mind to do so under hypnosis.

To be perfectly honest, I still wonder if it is possible. It is, however, logical that if the unconscious mind can turn down the metabolism (I have no doubt that it can) to keep a person from starving to death, then the unconscious mind has the ability to turn up the metabolism to produce more energy or warmth. At any rate, it is a simple thing to achieve under hypnosis, and it seems to work for my clients. The unconscious mind cannot think critically or distinguish fact from fantasy, so it's likely that the unconscious mind will uncritically accept the suggestion of speeding up the metabolism in the same way it accepts other suggestions under hypnosis.

The fourth thing that I do is give suggestions for deep breathing. One of the most energizing and cleansing things that you can do for your body is to practice deep breathing. You already know how to breathe deeply, and you can do these exercises virtually anytime and anywhere. There is no special equipment needed, and you can practice whether you have one minute available or 15 minutes. Deep breathing also relieves stress and can serve as a cue for you to slow down or concentrate. Controlled deep breathing can also increase the strength and power that you have available at any given moment.

Yoga, martial arts, tai chi, and many meditation practices have long recognized and documented the healthy benefits of deep breathing. One of the benefits is to speed up your metabolism.

The fifth suggestion that I give is to increase the amount of water that a person drinks. Water not only cleanses the body, it also energizes and speeds up the metabolism.

Suggestion: I can feel a very pleasant warming sensation beginning to course through my body. My metabolism is becoming heightened. I can feel the warmth caressing my skin. I can feel it spreading through my arms and legs. I can experience the pleasure of this sensation and the joy of having so much more energy to accomplish so many things. As my metabolism heightens more and more, I experience a surge of energy and motivation, enabling me to enjoy moving my body briskly in my preferred exercise. As my body pleasantly warms, I can imagine my extra pounds simply melting away. I can concentrate on raising my metabolism and feeling the wonderful warmth at any time at all. I enjoy this mental exercise, and I enjoy accelerating my weight loss more and more each and every day.

Habit 7. Exercise regularly

When you begin to lose a great deal of weight, is important that you do not lose muscle. Your goal should be to increase muscle while losing fat. These two things can and should be done simultaneously.

When developing an exercise habit, it is important to build on success. Your goals should be easily obtainable at first and gradually become more challenging. *Nothing motivates like success.* Suggestions are given to the clients to increase their levels of physical activity. Since the level of activity has been low and the energy level is low, I start with a low expectation for exercise. The suggestion might be for the client to walk 15 minutes per day at least three times a week and to begin *enjoying* walking more than before.

The increase in exercise gives a slight increase in energy, which can lead to more exercise and more energy. Twenty minutes of brisk walking can speed up the metabolism for hours.

As you become lighter and fitter, you will most likely be encouraged to develop muscle tone. The most effective way of doing this is by engaging in a weight lifting routine. It is beyond the scope of this book to deal with the specifics of weightlifting. There are a multitude of good books on the subject if you are interested in researching this for yourself. If you don't have the time or inclination to do the research—or even if you do—the services of a good personal fitness trainer can be very helpful.

Suggestion: As I follow my weight loss program, I begin to discover that I enjoy exercising my body. It feels so good to move my body rhythmically as I walk, or run, or swim, or do the treadmill, exercise bike, or (insert whatever type of exercise is most appealing to you). I like increasing the warmth of my body until I can enjoy the pleasant glistening of perspiration caressing my skin. It feels good to know that I am elevating my metabolism and that I will benefit from the after-burn of extra calories long after I am through exercising. Each and every step I take brings me closer to my goals. I know with each and every step I take, I am becoming leaner, fitter, healthier, and more attractive. The more I exercise, the easier it becomes, because my physical condition improves with every exercise session. It feels as if I enter a place of time distortion and 20 minutes of exercise begins to feel as if it is only 10 minutes. After I move my body continually for a few minutes, I discover my second wind and then I can exercise tirelessly for extended periods of time.

To develop your personalized hypnosis weight loss script: (A) Select an induction from the back of the book, (B) Include the suggestions listed here, and (C) Record the induction and your personalized script on a tape or CD. Listen to the tape each night as you drift to sleep. If you prefer you can simply order my weight loss CD. Again, instructions for ordering are included in the back of the book.

In addition to listening to your self-hypnosis tape each night, you should consciously learn each of the seven highly effective habits of thin people. Think about these habits each day. Write the habits down in your own handwriting, and post them by your bed.

Repetition is the mother of learning. The more frequently you remind yourself the sooner the seven highly effective habits of thin people will become automatic for you. Eventually—say after 28-33 days of you reminding yourself—you will master these seven habits.

If you are persistent in reminding yourself consciously, it will become second nature to quit eating when you are full. Think about it: *quit eating when you are full.* What a profound concept, and yet how many of us actually do this?

Now that you know and understand the seven highly effective habits of thin people, there is an action that you must take before they can become automatic in your life.

You must consciously decide to make these habits part of your conditioned responses.

8

Decide

When you have your plan in place, you must definitely **decide** to follow it. Decide means to cut off any other possibility. When you decide to lose 50 pounds, that decision should be irrevocable. You simply have to lose the weight; there is no other option. It has *got to be done because there are no other options.*

In the classic work *"The Art of War,"* Sun Tzu states that when your soldiers are frightened and poorly trained, and your enemy is brave and well trained; you can create a ferocious fighting force by placing your soldiers on killing ground. Using this strategy a general would march his troops into a boxed canyon where there is no retreat. The men would be ordered to let their horses go free and to break the wheels of their own wagons. The military leader would command that his ships be burned. The wise general would insure that there is no possible escape. The troops would be told that to retreat is not an option, the troops must conquer or perish. When an army of cowards knows that there is no way to live but to fight, they will fight with more ferocity than brave men. This is what the legendary Sun Tzu meant by: "placing your men on killing ground."

Former World Heavyweight Boxing Champion Muhammad Ali used to make such outrageous and boastful predictions that he would be totally humiliated if he lost. His boasting made it impossible for him even to consider defeat as an option.

If you are a person who is highly motivated by other people telling you can't do something, you can place yourself on killing ground by loudly and emphatically declaring that you will lose a definite number of pounds by a specific date. Invite skepticism and derision; welcome it as a challenge. Remember that "he who laughs last laughs best."

Because you *must* win this challenge, set it up so that you *will* win. As a general rule, calculate the weight loss at two pounds per week. If you have less than 30 pounds to lose, give yourself an extra three or four weeks because sometimes it may take the body three or four weeks to begin to release the weight. This is the phenomenon of homeostasis.

If you are the type of person who is discouraged by people telling you that you can't do something, then keep your intention private, telling no one but those persons who will support you. Even though the commitment that you make is a private one, tell yourself that your word to yourself is iron. "Honor is a gift a man gives himself."

9

Invest in yourself

The decision to invest in a hypnotist, a personal trainer, and/or a gym membership can be one of the wisest choices that you can make. It is interesting that people will willingly spend thousands on their wardrobe and medical insurance while balking at investing a few hundred dollars in their own physical appearance and good health.

Which would you rather be, an overweight person in an expensive dress or suit or a slender person in cheap jeans and a T-shirt?

When you think about it, the purchase of medical insurance is an investment in the possibility of your own poor health. You are essentially placing a wager that you will be in poor health. The insurance company is betting that you will be healthy. You only win that bet when you are in poor health. You win by losing. Doesn't it make sense to invest at least some money in the possibility of your vibrant health? In this instance, you win by winning. C'mon, think a happy thought, and go for the win!

Investing in yourself can be one of the most powerful things that you can do to increase your motivation and faith in yourself. When you spend money in support of your improvement, you say to yourself in a very powerful way that you believe in your own ability to achieve your dreams.

When I began to study hypnosis, my first thought was to continue to be a school principal until I retired. Then I would live on my retirement, and do hypnotherapy for free. Basically, I just wanted to help people, and I didn't feel good about taking their hard-earned money.

When I expressed this ambition to my professor, he was horrified. He explained it to me like this: "Lance you have an incredible aptitude for hypnosis. You have the ability to help people in very powerful ways, but if you do not charge for your services you will help no one. You will do yourself, your clients, and hypnosis itself a grave disservice.

People do not value what is given for nothing. A person's investment in herself is integral to the change or therapeutic process. A person who is willing to invest in herself is a very high functioning person. This type of person is leveraged to change. This person can learn what you can teach."

My professor went on to tell me that Milton Erickson, possibly the best known and most influential of modern day hypnotists, required his clients to make a substantial investment in dollars. If they had no money, he might set for them a challenge to climb to the top of Squaw Mountain, in which case the investment was in time and energy.

Personally, I am convinced that hypnosis works best when a person makes an investment in time, effort, and money. If you bought this book you have made a small investment in money, but you committed yourself to making a larger investment in time which includes reading this book, thinking about it, and doing the exercises. If you came to me for weight loss therapy, your investment in money would be greater, but your investment in time would be much less. Nevertheless, the investment is essential to this change process.

All learning carries a price. Fortunately, the greatest bargain of all is education. I have been known to modestly state that I give at least 100 times more value than the amount of money that I charge.

How much is it worth to be healthier, to have more energy, to improve your quality of life, to look better, to have a better sex life, to do your job better, to be calmer, to become more peaceful, and to have a sharper mind? What would it be worth to live even *one* more year?

Investing money, time, and energy reinforces your commitment to lose the weight *now*. However, you should never go to a hypnotist, personal trainer, or nutritionist with the expectation that you can pay them to solve your problem. You are the athlete, and they are the coach. Investing in yourself is another log you throw on the fire of your desire to have your ideal body.

10

Persistence

Persistence is an essential factor in transmitting the desire to lose weight into real weight loss. Whenever people have achieved great success, look behind the success and you will find the quality of persistence.

Thomas Edison tried unsuccessfully 10,000 times to invent the light bulb. When he was asked if he was discouraged, his reply was: "Not at all, I discovered 10,000 ways *not to* invent the light bulb." Within every failure, lie the seeds of success.

In America today, we have been conditioned by the media to expect *immediate* success on the first try. The 48-Hour Diet promises that you will lose 10 pounds in 48 hours. It is bad marketing to mention that you will most likely regain those 10 pounds in the following 48 hours!

It is not really our fault that the media has done an outstanding job of convincing us that weight loss should be immediate. Why does the media want you to think that weight loss should be quick? It is just good marketing.

The media knows people want to buy things that are quick and easy. Marketing experts sell weight loss products that have a short-term beneficial effect; if you have tried prescription or herbal weight loss formulas, you have probably discovered that *they really do work*. They can actually decrease your appetite while increasing your energy and speeding up your metabolism, resulting in weight loss.

If you have ever used these products for any period of time, you know that the beneficial effects gradually desist. You may have found yourself having to take more and more of the product to get the same effect. You may have even known that there were health risks involved. However, you have also known that there are health risks involved with being overweight. You may have considered the drug usage as an acceptable risk. However, you probably discovered that you had to take larger and larger doses to get the same effect. Eventually, you came to realize that the drug or herb produced no effect at all.

From the marketing experts' perspective, weight loss products are almost perfect. The customer keeps buying larger amounts of the product, because it does not result in sustained weight loss over time, the marketing experts continue to develop new short-term weight loss products and sell to the same customers. Not having the inclination to do the research involved, I can only imagine how much Americans spend on these types of weight loss products each year. The media's message is always the same. Don't be persistent in your weight loss program; try the next new, improved, quick, and easy weight loss program that comes along. Don't worry; it comes with a money-back guarantee. You have nothing to lose but the extra weight.

Advertising-experts know that most people will not use their money back guarantee even if they hate the product. It costs very little to give a money-back guarantee, and it is very effective at the point of the sale. I once saw a magazine add offering to predict the sex of your baby for a five-dollar fee. The advertisement promised a money back guarantee if they happened to be wrong. It is pretty easy to see that the advertiser will get to keep 50 percent of the money just by the Law of Averages. Marketing experts have mastered this science to woo you into buying their products. The techniques would not bad if the products that they offered could really end your struggle with weight for life. The problem is these products only distract us from using our innate ability to solve our weight problem without the need to use any product at all.

The truth of the matter is, you do not need to *buy any products* to lose weight. Weight loss is not quick, but it doesn't have to be difficult either. **You can condition yourself, in as little as 30 days, to develop habits that will end your need ever to buy another weight loss product**.

The media does not want you to know this fact. I know it sounds like I subscribe to conspiracy theories, but the truth is, that you already have everything you need within in you to begin enjoying losing all the weight you desire and maintaining your body at that ideal weight throughout the rest of your life. In as little as thirty days, you can end your *struggle* with your weight forever.

The key word here is "struggle." You will need to maintain your new habits for life, but you can learn to link so much pleasure with these new habits that no struggle is required. You can eat the foods that you enjoy most in just the right amounts and still lose all the weight that you desire. The key to changing your habits will be your willingness to be persistent over the next 28 to 33 days.

Notice I have not promised that you will lose all the weight that you want to lose in the next 28-33 days, but if you are persistent in changing your habits, you will end the *struggle* to lose weight for life. Depending on how much weight that you wish to lose, it may take you a good deal longer to lose weight than 28-33 days. Two pounds per week is a fair estimate.

Persistence in weight loss does not mean perfection. Frequently, in my hypnosis practice, a week after a client's first session I will hear him or her say:

Client: I messed up badly.

Lance: What happened?

Client: I binged and ate all the wrong things Sunday, and I ate too much of them also. I am so disgusted with myself. It is just not working for me.

Lance: How did you eat Monday?

Client: Just like we talked about: small portions and I made good choices.

Lance: How did you eat Monday through Saturday?

Client: Just like Monday?

Lance: So the suggestions were working Monday through Saturday?

Client: Yes, I guess so.

Lance: So the suggestions worked 6 out of 7 days?

Client: Yes.

Lance: So you were successful about 86 percent of the time? That is not so bad is it? I consider 86 percent to be a pretty good success rate. I am very proud of you.

Client: Really?

Lance: Yeah, really! Do you want to learn how to use your Sunday experience to have an even higher success rate next week?

Client: Yeah.

Lance: How did you feel about your weight loss program when you were following the suggestions Monday through Saturday?

Client: I felt good about it. I felt kind of proud.

Lance: And how did you feel Sunday?

Client: I felt terrible, like I was self-sabotaging, like I blew everything for nothing. I really didn't even want all that food, but I ate it anyway. I felt tired, bloated, sluggish, and like a big fat loser.

Lance: I am going to do you a big favor and help you remember that terrible feeling that you had Sunday.

Client: Gee, thanks! I can't believe I am paying you for this.

Lance: It is okay—you will thank me later. If you ever try to eat as badly as you did Sunday, simply tell yourself that you can eat any food you want in any amount. Then simply ask yourself if it is worth feeling like you felt Sunday. If you decide that it is, then eat another bite, chew it carefully, enjoy the taste, and ask yourself if it's really worth feeling the way you felt Sunday. If you still think it is—eat one bite at a time and persistently ask yourself: "Is it worth it?" I think you will discover that you simply lose interest in eating foods that are wrong for you.

One of the biggest problems in weight loss is the loss of motivation when we eat too much or make poor choices about the kinds of foods that we eat. People have a common tendency to want to quit when they have made a mistake. You can learn to use that experience of making a mistake to motivate yourself to do better in the future. Each mistake should serve as another log to fuel the fire of your desire to lose weight.

You will understand that improvement in weight management is never a straight line. It is a wiggly line with ups and downs, and this variation is totally acceptable as long as the highs are higher than the previous highs, and the lows are higher than the previous lows.

The trick is not to be discouraged by temporary failure. When you begin this weight loss program, you will discover that the rewards for complying with the program are both immediate and far-reaching. The negative consequences for noncompliance are also both immediate and far-reaching. Because in both instances the consequences are immediate, you will find it more pleasurable to comply than not to comply. This compulsion is the magic of this program, and it brings us to our next chapter on the pain and pleasure principles of human motivation.

11

Pain and Pleasure Principles of Human Motivation

I believe the two main motivators of human behavior are: (1) the need to avoid pain and (2) the desire to gain pleasure. Many people will say that love is a great motivator and it is not offered to gain pleasure or to avoid pain. I agree with the preceding statement, but I also know that when you do a selfless act motivated by unconditional love, you *will* feel pleasure. One can argue that the selfless act was not motivated by the desire to gain pleasure. However, because pleasure is a natural occurring consequence of giving love unconditionally it is difficult to determine that pleasure is not the motivator. In all other instances of human motivation it is clear that the need to avoid pain, or the desire to gain pleasure are the motivators of human behavior. Take a moment to think about this. See if you can establish another reason why we humans do the things that we do.

Assuming that you agree with the previous statement, we have a very clear way to look at the area of human motivation, especially as it applies to weight loss. If you are overweight, it is because you either associate more pleasure with those behaviors that create your weightiness; or you associate more pain with establishing new habits that will allow you to become your ideal weight and size. For most people, it is a combination of the two associations.

If it is really that simple, then the solution is also very simple. All we have to do is associate a great deal of pleasure with being our perfect weight and size. Then we associate massive amounts of pain with being overweight. Though it might surprise you, these associations are easily established when you understand how associations are made in the first place.

The problem is that we don't get an owner's manual with our brain, and we have collectively misunderstood how our brains work. To quote Will Rogers: "It is not what we don't know that hurts us. It is what we do know that ain't so."

In order for us to understand how associations are made in the first place, it is necessary to have some knowledge about brain theory. We have both a conscious and an unconscious mind. Some scientists estimate that about 20 percent of the things that we do are done with our conscious mind, and about 80 percent of the things that we do are controlled by our unconscious mind. Being a hypnotist, I think a more accurate split would be 10 percent conscious and 90 percent unconscious, but I will not argue the point. The important thing to know is the unconscious mind is bigger and stronger than the conscious mind.

Some of the things that we do with our conscious mind include using language, problem solving, and using logic. Right now you are using your conscious mind to read these words and determine if they make sense.

Some of the things that your unconscious mind controls are your breathing, your circulatory system, your digestive system, the growth of your skin, hair, and nails, your cells fighting an infection, etc. It has been estimated that between 1 million and 16 million processes are controlled by the unconscious mind every second—I am talking *every second*.

Essentially, our conscious minds are deletion-oriented. To explain this concept, I am going to introduce the term "field of awareness." By field of awareness, I mean everything that we *can choose* to see, smell, touch, taste, or hear at this moment is part of our field of awareness. Look around you. At this very moment, there are many *more* things in your field of awareness to which you can choose to attend than you *actually can* attend to consciously. In order to read this book you have to ignore almost everything else that comes into your field of awareness. (At least at the conscious level.)

For example, if you pay attention to the pictures on the wall, you would be unable to read this book at the same time. Although thoughts in the conscious mind may be changing very quickly, the conscious mind can still really only attend to one thing at a time. Everything else is simply deleted.

Yet as humans, we are required to do a great variety of things at the same time. If the conscious mind can only attend to one thing at a time, how do we accomplish this?

Let me give an example. Let us assume that you are trying to learn to drive a standard shift car. You would have to think consciously to move the stick to first gear while pushing in on the clutch, and then you would tell yourself to ease up on the clutch slowly while pushing on the accelerator.

If you are like most of us, the first few times you tried these coordinated actions, the car would lurch badly and die. Eventually, if you continue to practice, you get to the point where you can drive your car through traffic while listening to the radio and talking on the cell phone. Who knows? You might even be able to eat a cheeseburger at the same time. (But hopefully only if you're sufficiently underweight!)

As a matter of fact, if you drive a standard shift car long enough, you may find that when you drive an automatic car your hand is automatically moving to shift gears even though the action is quite unnecessary. The shifting behavior has become a *conditioned response* which means you don't think about it consciously; you just do it *automatically!*

Once the conscious mind, being the boss, has taught this gear-shifting behavior to the unconscious mind, it is then delegated to be one of the many millions of things that the unconscious mind can control simultaneously. When the conscious mind delegates this responsibility it becomes free to think analytically about the next problem that comes along.

We think that we go through life making many choices in each moment, but actually most of the things that we do are decided by conditioned response. Conditioned responses always have a trigger. A trigger sets a certain response in motion. A conditioned response also has an anchor. An anchor is that part of the response that experiences pleasure and thereby motivates the unconscious mind to repeat the conditioned response. Remember, central to human motivation is the desire to gain pleasure.

Thus we find that anytime the conscious mind has to deal with a mundane repetitive task, it will teach this task to the unconscious mind and delegate responsibility for carrying out the designated activity. Once the conscious mind has completed the delegation of the task, the unconscious mind takes over and the ensuing response becomes unconscious or automatic. The *unconscious mind is now in control of the activity.* Since the conditioned response has become automatic, the conscious mind will now have to use conscious effort, or willpower, to overcome that conditioning.

The conscious mind is capable of taking control of a conditioned response at any moment. However, the instant the conscious mind quits using energy or effort to control the conditioned response, the automatic conditioning will take over and direct the behavior. Using willpower is like pedaling a bicycle up a hill. A conditioned response is like gravity. The moment that you quit pedaling the bicycle up the hill, gravity begins to take over, and you begin to roll down the hill.

The first repetitive mundane task that we have to learn as infant humans is to breathe. Do you have to remind yourself to breathe? Of course not, this act has become unconscious and automatic. The second repetitive mundane task that we have to learn in order to survive is to eat. This is the seat of the problem with regard to weight loss: *eating has become an unconscious act. Eating has become automatic, a conditioned response under the control of the unconscious mind!* The pull to eat unconsciously has become like the pull of gravity.

Let me give you an example of how a conditioned response might work. Let us assume that you are a four-year-old child, and your mother has given you a chore to complete, such as cleaning your room. You work very hard and do a good job. Your mother rewards you by baking you all the cookies that you can eat. You feel proud of yourself, and the fresh cookies taste great. You associate *pleasure* with completing the task of cleaning the room. If this experience is repeated enough times, it will become a conditioned response.

In this scenario, doing a good job of finishing a task has become the trigger. Eating the cookies has become the anchor, and these components together create an unconscious conditioned response. As an adult, whenever you do a good job and complete a task (trigger), you may find that you experience a strong desire for cookies (anchor) that could be generalized to any sweet food that you enjoy.

You finish a project, and you eat some sweet, fattening food. You do all of this at an unconscious level because it has become a conditioned response. Even when you realize at the conscious level that this habit of rewarding yourself with sweets is causing you to be seriously overweight, putting you at risk for health problems, sapping your energy, reducing your productivity at work, causing you to be unattractive, and severely depressing your enjoyment of a normal sex life-even when you understand the negative consequences consciously, you seem to be powerless to change your behavior.

Why? Because once your conscious mind allows a conditioned response to occur, the conditioned response becomes more powerful than the conscious mind. Another word we could use for the conscious mind is your willpower. Another word we can use for the unconscious mind is your imagination. ₁*Whenever imagination and willpower come into conflict, eventually imagination will always win!* Why? The reason is the unconscious mind-or imagination is bigger (80 percent) and stronger, and it never sleeps.

To give you an example of the conflict between the conscious mind (willpower) and the unconscious mind (imagination), let us assume that you wish to kill yourself by using your willpower to hold your breath until you die. You use willpower to hold your breath. If your willpower is very strong you might be able to hold your breath until you become unconscious, then your imagination takes over and breathes. The fact is you cannot kill yourself by holding your breath no matter how hard you try.

Trying to lose weight by using your conscious mind (willpower) is like trying to kill yourself by holding your breath. You may be able to use your conscious mind to lose weight for a while, but eventually your imagination will take over.

Let us assume that you discover that your high school sweetheart is going to your 20-year class reunion. You become highly motivated to lose weight, and you use your willpower to do so. You simply tell yourself that you are not going to eat. You want to eat, but you don't because you are maintaining control of your eating through the active use of your willpower. You begin to lose weight through the use of your willpower.

Then you discover that your high school sweetheart is not coming after all. You become disappointed, or another way to say this is you experience emotional pain. Remember: central to human motivation is *the need to avoid pain.* You associate your efforts to lose weight with her not coming to the reunion. This association is so conditioned that every time you think of weight loss you think of her, and you experience pain.

You lose the will to lose weight. Think about losing weight is just too painful. Basic to human motivation is the need to avoid pain. Thinking about her equals pain. Thinking about losing weight equals pain. Basic to human motivation is the *need to avoid pain*! You can avoid pain by thinking about something else. *Humans have the power to choose their thoughts.*

You can choose to use your active imagination to think about something else. It is likely that you have a conditioned response that says whenever you feel emotional pain, think about eating some sweet and tasty food. Now you are thinking about eating chocolate ice cream (the desire to gain pleasure), and you aren't thinking of her or weight loss (the need to avoid pain). This conditioned response is automatically set in motion by the trigger of experiencing disappointment or emotional pain. The imagination takes control, creating images of how much immediate pleasure (anchor) you can gain by eating chocolate ice cream. You regain all the weight you lost, plus some extra pounds.

Perhaps you know for sure that your high school sweetheart is coming. You are motivated by your desire to gain the pleasure of seeing her see how good you look. This becomes a compelling image in your imagination, and you stay motivated and get to your perfect weight and size. Then you go to the reunion, and you find that she has gained 200 pounds. Now you are disappointed at how bad she looks. This disappointment creates emotional pain. Remember: emotional pain is the trigger for the conditioned response of eating chocolate ice cream. You regain all the weight you lost, plus some additional pounds.

Maybe your sweetheart is still a slender fox, and you have an amazing night with her, but then she leaves and so do you. Now you are separated from this vision of loveliness, separated by a great distance. You experience emotional pain, which is the trigger for you-know-what. You eat the ice cream and regain all the weight that you lost, plus some extra pounds.

You may marry your high school sweetheart, but then she becomes bossy, demanding, and hypercritical. This creates emotional pain. Which triggers what? You guessed it: you gain back all the weight that you lost, plus some extra pounds.

Let's face it: life is full of emotional pain. As long as you have this emotional pain trigger a conditioned response to eat ice cream, you aren't going to stay slender. It simply will not happen. This is what the struggle of losing weight is all about, and this is why at least *65 percent of all Americans are losing this struggle.* We are fighting a battle that our biological nature will not allow us to win. To win this battle is like trying to stand on your own shoulders; your physiology will not allow this to happen. So what is the solution?

The good news is that the solution is very, very simple. All we have to do is change this conditioned response to eat mass quantities of fattening food when you experience emotional pain to a better, more empowering conditioned response. In this book, you will learn how to change that conditioned response to something that enables you to maintain the lifestyle of a slender, healthy, and happy person.

What I am saying is, at some point your imagination will kick in and overpower your willpower. *When imagination and willpower come into conflict, imagination will always eventually win.* Remember: your imagination is bigger, stronger; and it never sleeps.

Tony Robbins has said it and Dr. Phil has said it, and now I am saying it. Ninety-five percent of the people who go on a diet and actually lose weight regain all the weight that they lost within two years and gain some additional weight as well.

To my mind, the interesting thing about these studies is that the 5 percent of people who maintained their weight loss all learned to think about food in a different way, using their *imagination* to associate massive amounts of pleasure with being their ideal weight and size. In other words, they changed their conditioned responses at the *unconscious level.*

When someone tells me, "I just can't lose weight; I have no willpower," I say, "That is great because we are not going to use willpower; we are going to use *imagination.*" Whenever imagination and willpower come into conflict, imagination is the winner and willpower is the loser, and I will make that bet every single time.

So where do conditioned responses come from? Would it surprise you to know that far and away most of our conditioned responses are established before we reach the age of five or six? It is absolutely true, and what is more amazing is that most of our conditioned responses have no real rhyme or reason to them. They are just randomly paired neural-associations.

In 1904, a Russian scientist named Pavlov won the Nobel Peace prize for his experiments with dogs. He would ring a bell and then present food, ring a bell and present food. He repeated this many times. Eventually the dogs began to associate food with the bell, and they began to salivate. Even when they rang the bell and no food was presented, the dogs began to salivate just as if food had actually been presented.

One thing Pavlov established is that when two unrelated stimuli are repeatedly paired together, an association or a conditioned response is created in the unconscious mind. It doesn't have to be logical or make sense. Pavlov could have blown a whistle, clapped his hands, or just hummed Dixie and presented food, and the association would have been made. Subsequent research has proven that this conditioned response process is the same in humans as it is in dogs.

Getting back to where conditioned responses come from: Before we reach the age of about five or six we pretty much uncritically accept into our conscious mind everything that we hear. This accounts for the amazing rapidity with which small children learn. If you are three or four years old and your father says, "That man over there is Santa Claus," you are probably going to believe it. If you find 50 cents under your pillow and your mother says in an excited voice that the tooth fairy was there, you are probably going to believe it.

However, somewhere around the age of five or six, we begin to realize that people don't always tell us the truth, and we begin to develop a critical filter. Every time you are lied to, mislead, tricked, or taken snipe hunting, this critical filter becomes thicker. This filter is necessary for our protection. Without it, people would cheat us and take advantage of us. We would be too suggestible. We would buy every product advertised on television. If someone invited us to rob a liquor store, we would simply hop in the car and go.

By the time that we get to be adults, this filter has become so thick that 99 percent of what we hear is not accepted into our unconscious mind. This is why most of what we do is driven by conditioned responses developed during our early childhood.

Now let us revisit the same scenarios presented above, but this time we will change the conditioned response to one that empowers us to lose weight. Once again, we find that our high school sweetheart is coming to the reunion, and again we are highly motivated to lose weight. Alas and alack, we discover that she is not coming after all. Once again, we experience emotional pain. Once again this serves as a trigger to put our conditioned response into automatic action, *ah, but this time the conditioned response is different.*

The new conditioned response is: whenever I experience emotional pain from not having something that I desire, I develop a plan to do what I can to fulfill my desire, I take action, and follow my plan. As long as I follow my plan, I experience pleasure because I am getting closer to my goal.

In other words, I have determined in my imagination that I can still have what I want if I will make a good plan and stick to it. Remember: the unconscious mind has no ability to distinguish fact from fantasy. So whether or not this conditioned response is true, your unconscious mind will accept it as truth. *Humans have the ability to choose their thoughts! Why not choose thoughts that empower us?* If I am dying of thirst and I see a glass of water, what is important is not whether the water is real, but whether it will refresh me. Will it quench my thirst?

In this scenario, the emotional pain of not seeing her triggers the new conditioned response to develop a plan so that you can still see your high school sweetheart. You then decide to take action and develop a plan. You do this automatically. It has become part of your basic nature.

Your new plan could be to drive down and see her. Remember: according to your response, it doesn't necessarily have to be a good or logical plan. As long as it is a plan and you are following it, the action of following your plan will register as pleasurable in your unconscious mind.

The action of following the plan has become the *anchor*. Your plan could be to (1) to lose all the weight you desire and (2) drive down and see her. In this instance, you might be even more motivated to lose the weight because you are going to all the trouble and potential embarrassment to see her. So you are motivated to lose weight because you know that you are definitely going to see her.

Maybe you drive down to see her, you look great, and she is very impressed. You have a wonderful time. You experience the anchor (all that pleasure), and your conditioned response is strengthened.

Perhaps you drive down to see her, she has gained 200 pounds, and she is no longer your heart's desire. I know this is shallow, but it could happen! There are no guarantees in life. In this case, you may experience disappointment or emotional pain, which triggers your conditioned response developing a plan to gain something else that you want. Once again, you associate pleasure with following your plan.

You may decide to drive down to see her, and you look great but she still isn't impressed, and she doesn't want to be around you. Hey, there are no guarantees, it could happen! In this scenario you experience emotional pain, which triggers your conditioned response to think of a plan to get what you want. Maybe you think, if I get rich then she will want me. So you think of a plan to get rich, and you follow it until you are rich.

I am not telling you to do things to impress other people, for this may not be the best conditioned response available for you. The point is with this new conditioned response, your outcomes are much different. In the first scenario, you lost all the weight you wanted to lose and you were rewarded with massive amounts of pleasure. In the second scenario, you lost all the weight that you wanted to lose. You just changed your ultimate goal. In the third scenario, you lost all the weight you wanted to lose, plus you got rich as well.

I am not telling you that you have to behave in this manner, I am just saying the results you got drastically changed because your conditioned response was different. I know this type of conditioned response is possible because I have done this for myself. I have established a conditioned response, which says there is always a way to get what you want if you are really committed. By the way, this is not even a conditioned response that I invented. I heard Tony Robbins say this was a belief that he had. I liked it, and I stole it. Actually, I paid for the CD series so I don't think that I can be arrested. What I am saying is if you hear of a belief that you like, it is possible using the technology presented in this book to turn that belief into a conditioned response at the automatic thinking level of your brain.

This belief has allowed me to turn massive amounts of emotional pain into enthusiasm, energy, and challenges. Remember: as long as I am improving and moving in the direction of my goals, I am experiencing pleasure. It really does feel good. *You can choose your thoughts, so why not choose thoughts that empower you? Why not choose thoughts that make you feel good?*

If you are experiencing any powerful negative or positive emotion, I challenge you to harness that energy to drive you to complete a goal that is worthwhile, maybe something like losing all the weight that you desire. It worked for me, and it can work for you. Any powerful emotion that you can experience can drive you to move in the direction of your goal. *Never waste emotional energy; it is more valuable than gold. No matter how negative that it might appear to be at the time, it can always be harnessed to achieve some worthwhile goal, and it sure beats wallowing in negativity, depression, and self-pity.* I will talk more about this in the chapter on harnessing the power of your emotions.

In summary, humans are motivated by just two things: (1) the need to avoid pain and (2) the desire to gain pleasure. Most of our behaviors are a result of conditioned responses and these responses have become automatic. A trigger is pulled, firing the conditioned response gun.

Because these responses are under the control of the unconscious mind, efforts to control them consciously will always ultimately fail. This would be like trying to open the garage door with the television remote control. Instead of trying to control the conditioned response with the conscious mind or willpower, it makes much more sense to simply change the conditioned response. Once the conditioned response is changed to a more empowering one, the behavior changes *automatically and without conscious effort!*

The question remains, how do we change our conditioned response? There are a number of ways to do this. In my opinion, the quickest, easiest, and most effective way is through the application of the scientific principles of hypnosis.

12

Hypnosis

Any scholar with an open mind will readily admit that the historical documentation proving that hypnosis works is overwhelming. The sleep temples of ancient Egypt date back to 1,000 B.C. These "temples" were places where priests put worshippers to "sleep" and suggested that they be cured and they usually were. These temples were so successful and lucrative that they were established in ancient Greece and Rome as well.

A Greek engraving from 928 B.C. shows Chiron, the most renowned physician of his time, placing his pupil Aesculapius under hypnosis. In 1773, Anton Messmer began curing thousands of people in the French Court using the power of suggestion. Documentation of the successful use of hypnosis by such notables as The Marquis De Puysegur, Father Gasner, Dr. James Braid, Burco, and Charcot fill the pages of history.

This is a very brief scanning of the history of hypnosis, but this book is not about proving that hypnosis works. It is about the practical application of hypnosis and related technologies to allow you to enjoy losing all the weight that you desire to lose.

In summary, for thousands of years mankind has known that hypnosis works. For a long time, we simply did not understand the scientific principles that explain *why* it works. Unfortunately, the lack of understanding about the true nature of hypnosis has led to a number of myths that have been associated with it. The good news is we now have the technology to prove why and how the science behind hypnosis works.

Just as there have been major breakthroughs in computers and wireless communication in the last 30 years, the breakthroughs in understanding how our brain works have been just as dramatic. Scientist now know that there is electrical energy in our brains, and science has labeled brain states based on measures of this electrical energy, which can be measured by an EEG machine.

We know for instance that if you are in a conscious mind state, the scientific name for that state of mind would be Beta, and it means that your brainwaves are moving at a rate of approximately 33 cycles per second. If you allow yourself to drift into a light state of hypnosis, your brainwaves will be in a state called Alpha. The rotation of your brain waves will be approximately 14 cycles per second. If you drift into Theta or deep hypnosis, your brainwaves slow down to approximately 7 cycles per second. If you drop into a very deep sleep, known as Delta, your brainwaves will slow down to approximately 4 Cycles Per Second.

In the last chapter, I talked about what the critical filter does. In this chapter, I will explain *how* it works. This knowledge is vital to understanding the scientific principles of hypnosis. You may remember from the previous chapter that up until about the age of five or six, children uncritically accept into their unconscious minds almost everything that they hear. At the age of about five or six, they begin to realize that people don't always tell them the truth. At the age of five or six most children begin to develop a critical filter that serves to filter out information that the conscious mind believes to be untrue. You might remember that I estimated that by the time we get to be adults, we generally do not accept into the unconscious mind 99 percent of the things that we hear. The question is: how does the critical filter work?

You can think of the critical filter as being like a ceiling fan. Imagine or visualize, if you will, a ceiling fan rotating at a very high speed. When you look up at that fan, the blades are rotating so fast that the fan appears to be solid. You cannot see empty space between the fan blades. If you get above the ceiling fan and try to drop a pencil through the blades of the fan, the pencil will be rejected.

You simply cannot drop the pencil through, but if you were able to slow that fan down by more than half speed, let us say slow it down from Beta (conscious state, 33 cycles per second) to Alpha (light hypnosis, 14 cycles per second), then you could see empty space between the blades, and more importantly, you could time the drop of the pencil *through* the fan. If you slowed the fan down even further to Theta (deep hypnosis, 7 cycles per second), it would be even easier to drop that pencil through.

Think of the fan as the critical filter, hypnosis through progressive relaxation as the speed control on the fan, and the pencil is the suggestion. When the suggestion is accepted into the unconscious mind, a new conditioned response or habit is born. *Remember: the unconscious mind has no ability to think critically. When you get a suggestion past the critical filter, it will be accepted uncritically.* Much the same as when a baby is conceived, the body doesn't ask whether or not it should be born; it simply accepts the conception and makes the baby.

When we get past the critical filter, we return to that innocent childlike state of hyper-suggestibility. In this innocent state you will accept the suggestion; the suggestion creates the new conditioned response. Walla! The new baby is born!

It is important to note that a new conditioned response or habit is like a baby. It is weak and fragile in the beginning. It will need to be nurtured and fed in order to grow into a big, and powerful conditioned response. A new conditioned response is most vulnerable during the first 28 to 33 days of its life. If it lives past this point, its chance of growing into a big, powerful, self-sustaining habit increases exponentially. Hypnosis through progressive relaxation gives a painless birth to this new baby habit, but what will the habit need in order to grow?

The food that this baby habit will eat is imagination. The baby will need exercise or repetition to grow strong. Just as a human baby must experience love to thrive, a baby habit must experience pleasure. *Remember: the basic motivations of human behavior are the need to avoid pain and the desire to gain pleasure.* The new habit will need to have both of these conditions met. Pleasure will *serve as the anchor that reinforces the response. Pleasure is the catalyst of the development of a new habit.*

When you think about it, raising a baby does not entail a lot of hard physical labor, but *it is very demanding.* You wouldn't dream of leaving an infant unattended for very long because that infant is dependent on you to fulfill his needs. We attend to our children for a while, and, with any luck, there comes a time when our children grow up into strong independent adults who cannot only attend to their own needs but can attend to our needs as well. Think of your new conditioned response as a child who will, with proper care and in short order, grow up and take care of you–*automatically!*

The good news is that it doesn't take a generation to raise a new conditioned response, if properly reared, a new conditioned response will take care of your needs. On that premise you have my personal guarantee. If you follow the recipe presented here, you *will* lose all the weight that you desire.

Hypnosis, as I have just described, is the result of a relaxation induction. The most commonly used induction is a progressive relaxation induction. I have included several progressive relaxation inductions in the back of this book. You can choose one that appeals to you and read it into a tape recorder. Then read the suggestions in the back of the chapter into the recorder after the induction has been read. Remember to speak in a deep, soothing, rhythmic fashion, saying each word clearly and distinctly, or you can have a friend read the induction to you as you close your eyes and relax. If you wish, you can simply order my weight loss compact disc or contact me for a personal session.

Progressive relaxation is only one method of hypnosis, but it is the least misunderstood. It is very effective for weight loss. It is beyond the scope of this book to give a complete discussion of hypnosis. This book is essentially not about hypnosis but about weight loss. You can effectively lose weight by reading this book and following the principles listed with or without hypnosis. Hypnosis is just one very powerful weapon that can be used in the "battle of the bulge."

Hypnosis is just one of many tools that I intend to share with you for your consideration. You will have the freedom to choose those techniques that are most appealing to you.

I have often thought that if clients would read this book before our first session, the therapy would be even stronger than it is. Ideally, a client would read the book and then come in for weight loss hypnotherapy. There is simply not enough time for me to present all the information presented in this book during a session.

In summary, the validity of hypnosis can be proven both historically and via scientific technology. Hypnosis works because it allows suggestions to get past the critical filter into the unconscious mind. Hypnosis gives birth to the new habit, but that habit must be nurtured in order to survive.

Throughout the remainder of this book, you will be given practical tools to lose all the weight that you desire and to maintain that weight-loss for life. The end results: your habits will *automatically* keep you slender, fit, attractive, and healthy, with a greater zest for and enjoyment of life. In short, you will avoid the pain of being overweight and enjoy the pleasure of being your ideal weight and size.

13

Auto Suggestion

Through the use of the principles of autosuggestion, the conscious mind can transfer messages to the unconscious mind. Because the unconscious mind is bigger and stronger, when transferring a thought from the conscious mind, the thought becomes more powerful. It can become automatic.

Dominating thoughts in the conscious mind voluntarily reach the unconscious mind and become a part of the mind's automatic thinking process. In order to achieve your goal you should permit only those thoughts that serve your best interests to *dominate in your conscious mind*!

If the dominating thought in your mind is: I can't quit eating; I just can't control my eating. The principle of autosuggestion will work, this thought will be transferred to your unconscious mind, and your eating will be automatic and out of control. However, the same thought process that has caused you to be overweight could be used to empower you to lose weight.

If the dominating thought in your mind is, nothing tastes as good as thin feels. This thought will transfer to your unconscious mind and become an automatic part of your thinking process.

The key to using autosuggestion is really very simple. Allow your best thoughts to dominate. The problem is, we already have established dominating thoughts in our conscious mind. If you are overweight, it is certain that you think thoughts that cause you to behave in ways that cause you to be overweight. Unless you are actively using your conscious mind to choose positive thoughts, negative ones will occur. Your mind is like a garden plot. You can choose what kind of plants to grow in that garden, but if you fail to choose, weeds will grow there automatically.

If you want to grow roses, you are going to have to plant roses, water, weed, and tend to those roses. You can think of the principles of autosuggestion as a handbook for gardening the mind.

You must first decide what thoughts you desire to dominate in your mind. For example, let us plant the following thoughts: I enjoy eating smaller portions of food. Food is becoming less and less important to me now. I find myself drawn to healthy, nutritious foods that are high in protein and low in carbohydrates, and I find myself losing the desire to eat foods that are not good for me.

These are the varieties of flowers that you have planted in your mind. Next you will need to water these flowers. Emotion is the water that the flowers of the mind must have in order to thrive or even survive. The thoughts will only grow if they are mixed well with emotion. Plain, unemotional words do not influence the unconscious mind. You must learn to emotionalize your thoughts with belief. Faith, love, and sex are the strongest positive emotions that you can use. If you have experienced pain from being overweight, learn to re-experience that pain and pair that emotion with a positive thought from your mind.

For example, if you have ever wanted to be involved with someone romantically but that was not possible because of your weight and physical condition, re-experience the emotional pain. Associate that pain with eating fattening foods. If the association is made, you will have a need to avoid fattening foods.

Because of your weight, you are worried about your health, and you feel sad because you know you need to live to raise your grandchildren. You can imagine yourself dying from complications arising from morbid obesity, and your grandchildren being split up and taken to less desirable places to be raised. If you can imagine this until a tear comes to your eye, you can pair this emotion with the thought that food is becoming less and less important to you. Your health and physical well-being is becoming more and more important in your life.

If you can remember a time in your life when you were slender, re-experience all the joy associated with that picture in your mind's eye. See yourself that way, and *know* that you will absolutely be that way again.

Each person will be able to feel strong emotions in different ways. Don't get discouraged if you can't do it right away. Society teaches us to keep our emotions in check. We are not taught to use the strength of our emotions as nuclear fuel to power us in the direction of our goals. However, with persistence and practice, you will learn to use the power of your emotions to drive your daily actions until you reach your goal.

I am not saying that you need to make yourself an emotional basket case. I am merely suggesting that you find some time to do this exercise once a day. Go to some quiet place (preferably in bed at night) where you will not be disturbed or interrupted. Repeat out loud (so you may hear your own words) the amount of weight that you wish to lose and the exact date by which the weight definitely will be lost. Describe what you intend to do to gain this ideal body that you desire and deserve.

For example: By the first day of June, I will weigh 130 pounds. I will lose all the excess weight between now and then by changing my thoughts and behaviors with regard to eating and exercise. I will begin losing the weight now and will not stop until I reach my goal. I will plant good thoughts in the garden of my mind. I will water those thoughts with emotion. I will weed out all negative thoughts by focusing on the good thoughts, and I will attend to this garden with everlasting persistence.

Repeat this affirmation once in the morning and once upon going to bed. See yourself at your ideal weight and size. Place a written copy of this affirmation where you can read it each morning when you awake and each evening when you go to bed.

Next you must learn how to weed the negative thoughts from your mind. Remember: the conscious mind cannot attend to two separate thoughts at the same time. Whatever you think about becomes stronger in your life, and if you ignore a thought, it dies from lack of attention. *When a negative thought appears, think of an equivalent positive one.* For example, when the thought "I want to eat chocolate candy" appears, think of the thought "nothing tastes as good as thin feels." Whenever the thought to eat the candy appears, counter with the thought that nothing tastes as good as thin feels.

Think of the negative thought as being like a punch that you have learned how to block. Determine that you will continue to block the punches until they quit coming. You will find with a sense of amusement that you counter the attack every time. The thought can no longer penetrate because you know the defense. You are determined to defend as long as it takes. Imagine someone throwing a thousand punches at you with each punch effectively blocked; eventually the punches will quit coming. The positive thoughts will dominate.

Memorize a few affirmations. At the end of this book I have included a couple of pages of weight loss affirmations. Choose the ones that appeal most to you, and use them to counter every negative thought. Determine that you will counter every negative thought with a positive one.

14

The Power of Pretend

I remember pretending as a child. In those days, there were no video games, or soccer leagues, no VCRs, or DVDs, no movies to rent. When we played, we used our imaginations. If we played monster, one person was designated as the monster. The rest of us would scream in terror and flee as if that person were really a blood-sucking vampire. If I wanted to play cowboy, I could instantly turn a stick into a white stallion. My finger and thumb served effectively as a pistol. I could just as easily transform that stick into a sword, and suddenly I was Sir Lancelot fighting the evil Mordred. Looking back, I could use my imagination to do anything I wanted. I was almost God-like because I had mastered the power of pretend.

As the years went by, I was discouraged from using my imagination. My teachers scolded me for pretending; as I grew older the kids would begin to make fun of me for pretending. I began to use my pretend muscle less and less. My powerful pretend ability gradually began to diminish but my pretend muscles did not dissipate with age; they became diminished through lack of use. I didn't realize that I was giving up a very powerful strategy for ones that weren't as much fun and didn't work nearly as well.

I was taught to analyze the situation, to assess the odds, to make logical decisions by predicting statistical probabilities. It is my belief that if you use these types of strategies with regard to weight loss, you will have doomed yourself to be overweight, lethargic, inactive, and far less attractive than you can be. This method is just one more attempt to try to overcome the imagination by using the conscious mind. Remember: it is impossible to kill yourself by using your conscious mind to hold your breath because *whenever the conscious mind and the unconscious mind come into conflict, the unconscious mind will always win!*

For example, let us analyze the weight loss situation in America. In America today, 65 percent of the population is overweight, which means you have about a one in three chance of being slender. If this statistical fact does not put doubt in your mind and lessen your faith in your ability to lose weight, you have failed to grasp the concept of statistical probability. If that fact failed to discourage you, then this one should. Ninety-five percent of the people who actually go on diets and lose weight regain all the weight they lost plus some additional pounds within two years.

Statistics show that people become more overweight as they age. How is that for a happy thought? Do you know anyone who is currently not getting older? Talk about dumping water on your fire of desire to lose weight. Statistics is a very accurate and verifiable science. Statistics don't lie.

This may all be true, but I would like you to consider for a moment a cause and effect question. Are statistics accurate because people have little ability to influence the conditions of their lives or are they true because people know these statistics, and they tend to believe and repeat them until they become self-fulfilling prophecies? *What a person believes to be true usually does become true in his or her reality!*

In other words, if you buy into the concept that you are just another piece of flotsam tossed around on the sea of statistical probability, then you will fit into the statistical norm. Please consider this: it is also a statistical truth that the people who are slender are either not aware of the statistics, or they believe that they are not a part of the statistical norm. Because you can choose your thoughts, why not choose to believe that you can be a part of the 35 percent of the population who is not overweight?

Rediscover your power of pretend. Pretend that you are a part of the elite percentage who accomplishes their weight loss goals for life. Don't stop there. When you know you have eaten the right amount of food for you, pretend you are full. Let out a deep sigh, hold your belly and say, "Man am I full; I feel like I am about to explode; I couldn't eat another bite; I hope I can get up from the table."

Make a game out of trying to convince the people with whom you are eating that you are full. Pretend that you are a great actor, and you must convince everyone eating with you that you are full to the point of explosion. Watch the incredulous looks on their faces. Listen to their exclamations of disbelief. Note with a sense of amusement that they are incredulous at how you could be full after eating so little food. Have fun with it! *Pretending is fun!*

Explain to them that you have been reading this book, and you gave yourself a hypnotic suggestion. Ever since then you find that you get full after eating just the right amount of food. Explain to them that you have eaten to the point of perfect nutritional comfort and satisfaction, and you have given yourself a hypnotic suggestion that should you try to eat one bite past this point, you will have to endure the many negative consequences of overeating. Among these consequences is a bloated feeling that may lead to nausea. If they insist that you eat something else, pretend that you are stifling a gag reflex, excuse yourself from the table, and go to the rest room. Have a good laugh! Make a game out of it!

If you are persistent and consistent in your performance, you will find that they will begin to believe you. You will also find that if you practice this performance every time you eat, *eventually you begin to believe you.* You will actually become full when you have eaten the perfect amount of food for you. When you are pretending to be full, just remember to also pretend that you are not pretending that you really are full. You may want to pretend that you never pretended at all. It is all up to you, for you have 100 percent control over your power of pretend, and like any other muscle, it grows stronger the more you use it.

You might say that this would be deceptive to do to friends. I ask you to consider this statement: all skills, abilities, and accomplishments start out as pretend. The wolf puppy that will one day grow into a ferocious fighter starts out as a small puppy pretending to fight with his brothers and sisters. Is the same thing not true with every other mammal? Does the kitten not pretend to stalk and pounce upon his prey?

What do you think Michael Jordan, Troy Aikman, Emmitt Smith, Mark McGuire, Tiger Woods, or any other elite athlete did as a child? I would be willing to bet if you asked them they would say that they pretended to be the best at their respective sports. Much of their ability could be traced to the countless hours that they spent pretending to be great.

George Washington pretended to be a noble man. He pretended to be a gentleman, a soldier, and a great statesman. He pretended so successfully that he married into nobility, developed cultured manners, became commissioned as a General, and was elected President. You might say that all the revolutionary soldiers pretended that there was a country called the United States of America until one day the existence of this country became a reality.

Never underestimate the power of pretend. More importantly, use this pretend power to enable you to accomplish your goals. If you still think that this is a deceptive thing to do to your friends, consider this last point: *pretending is contagious!*

When I was in college, four or five of us would stand by a busy road and look into a tree. We would pretend that there was something very unusual and a little bit frightening in that tree. We would look up into the tree, point, and move back cautiously or laugh nervously. We coordinated our movements so that we moved at the same time. When one of us made a reaction, the rest of us would try to duplicate it. It was all for fun. It was all-pretend.

We found within a short time, dozens of people pulled their cars over and came to stare into the tree. We would ask them what they saw, and amazingly enough, some people actually described what they thought was an animal. Some figured out what we were doing, laughed heartily, and joined us in fooling the newcomers. Everyone left the tree feeling better than when they came. Some left with the belief that they had seen a truly strange and marvelous animal. Their lives had been enriched in some way.

The point of this story is: *the more people there are who pretend the easier it becomes to pretend.* If you pretend to be full in this convincing way, it will be easier for your friends to read this book, give themselves the hypnotic suggestions, and pretend as well. When you and your friends are sitting there, each of you at your perfect weight and size, feeling full of energy and self-confidence, looking and feeling better than you ever have; it will be an interesting point to ponder. Did I accomplish my weight loss goals through reading the book, affirmations, hypnosis, or through pretending? It will be an interesting point to ponder, but it won't really matter now, will it?

Here are some suggestions for using your power of pretend:

- Pretend that you don't like some fattening food that you once thought you liked.

- Pretend that in the past you only pretended to like a specific food that is bad for you, but all along you have actually hated the taste of it.

- Whenever you try to eat something that you know is bad for you, pretend that your taste buds have become so highly developed that you can now taste all the preservatives and chemicals in that food, and they taste terrible.

- Pretend that you enjoy exercising.

- Pretend that you prefer the taste of water to that of every other beverage.

- Pretend you are raising your metabolism, you can feel your body getting warmer, and you can feel your pounds melting away.

- Pretend that you are happy, relaxed, poised, and self-confident.

- Pretend that you are never hungry past 7 p.m.

- Pretend that you enjoy eating healthy and nutritious foods in just the right amounts.

- Pretend that you enjoy eating your food more slowly.

- Pretend that nothing tastes as good as thin feels.

- Pretend that you enjoy losing weight that it is a fun and exciting game-a game you are sure that you will win!

If you truly master the power of pretend, you will lose all the weight you desire to lose. The power of pretend can be used as an individual strategy or incorporated with the other techniques that I will share with you in this book. In the next chapter, you will learn how to utilize the power of questions.

15

The Power of Questions

Allow some time today to observe yourself. Allow yourself to become a bit emotionally detached for a short time. For 30 minutes or an hour, become a very objective observer. I think that you will discover that you are always asking yourself questions: Why did he say that? What is going on? What does that mean? So what am I going to do now? If she does that, what will I do?

I think that you will discover that questions like these are always going through your mind. We are constantly engaged in a conversation with ourselves, asking questions and trying to find the answers. Our mind functions by asking questions, evaluating questions, and coming up with answers. All evaluation is question-asking. The prefix of question is quest. By evaluating questions, our conscious mind decides what to do next. The questions that you ask yourself determine the focus of your thoughts. *Whatever you focus on consistently becomes stronger in your life.*

If you ask yourself a question with the sincere desire to receive an answer, your brain will come up with an answer. Even if the question has no basis in reality. An important law about questions is the *Law of Presupposition*. Many questions have presuppositions that are accepted uncritically by the unconscious mind. For instance, if you continually ask yourself, "Why can't I ever lose weight?" your conscious and your unconscious mind immediately accepts as fact that you cannot lose weight and gets busy coming up with reasons why you can't lose weight. This question undermines the very faith that is essential to the process of weight loss.

Your mind may say you can't lose weight because of genetics or thyroid problems, or because you eat continually, and you never exercise. It may come up with reasons like, "You have no self-control" or "You are trying to sabotage yourself." The point is, if you ask yourself a poor quality question, you get a poor quality response. You can learn to ask yourself better quality questions.

I am going to list a few questions that people frequently ask themselves about weight loss. See how many of these questions you have asked yourself:

- Why am I so fat?

- Why can't I lose weight?

- Why don't I have any self-control?

- Why do I love all the foods that are bad for me?

- Why do I always overeat?

- Why am I so lazy?

- Why can't I get motivated to lose weight?

- Why can't I control my eating?

- Why do I hate to exercise?

- Why is losing weight so hard?

You can see that each one of these questions presupposes failure, and even worse, they set your mind working on reasons to verify and justify your failure. Asking yourself these types of questions is like dumping sands on the fire of your desire to lose weight. The solution is very simple and painless. You can quickly and easily learn to ask better quality questions, questions that will feed and stoke the fire of your desire to lose weight. It is just as easy to ask questions that empower you to achieve your goal as it is to ask questions that sabotage your success.

Avoid using *why* questions, as they are open-ended questions that keep your mind busy coming up with endless possibilities that serve no positive purpose. I strongly suggest that you change your *why* questions to *how* questions.

When you ask a better quality question, that presupposition will become fixed in your mind. For example, when you ask yourself the question, "How will I lose all the weight I want to lose and enjoy the process?" Your unconscious mind presupposes that you can lose weight, and you can enjoy the process. Now the mind works on an answer. Your mind may make the connection that you enjoy playing tennis and that tennis is a good exercise that will help you to lose weight.

The answer might be to join a tennis league and play on a regular basis. Your mind will come up with a list of things that you enjoy and determine how enjoyment of those activities could possibly lead to weight loss. Do not underestimate your mind's ability to come up with a good answer for a good question. *You have the ability to come up with creative answers that are right for you.*

Any good question that you can design can motivate you to lose weight, but to keep it simple, I suggest you replace any negative question that you might have with regard to weight-loss with this one question: "How will I safely lose all the weight that I desire and enjoy the process?" This book alone will give you many answers to this question, and you will have utilized yet another powerful technique for imprinting into your unconscious mind the fact that *you can lose weight and enjoy the process.*

The summary for this chapter is extremely simple. Take note whenever you ask yourself a negative question about weight loss, and replace it with the question: How will I safely lose all the weight that I desire and enjoy the process?

16

The Law of Reverse Suggestion

One of the most powerful laws of hypnosis is the *Law of Reverse Suggestion*. Almost everyone who goes on a diet and tries to lose weight uses this principle of suggestion in a way that defeats one's ability to lose weight. It is my belief that almost all diets fail because people *use this principle in the wrong way*. Once you understand this very simple rule of human suggestibility, you can avoid making the mistake that almost everyone on a diet makes.

The Law of Reverse Suggestion is really very simple. To illustrate how the principle works: for the next 15 seconds, "***Don't think of a pink elephant!***" What did you think about? You had to think about a pink elephant in order to try not to think about it. It is like trying to look at the print on a page without reading the words. Once we learn to read we automatically decode the words that we see. When we learn language we automatically picture the words we hear.

Not only does the statement "***Don't think of a pink elephant***" not keep you from thinking of a pink elephant, it actually increases the likelihood that you will think of a pink elephant by approximately 100 percent. Further, the *Law of Reverse Suggestion will actually intensify and strengthen the suggestion*. For example, of the two suggestions "***Please think of a pink elephant and don't think of a pink elephant***," the second suggestion is actually the strongest.

More mental energy is expended on trying not to think about it than on trying to think about it. In order not to think about a pink elephant, you have to hold the thought of a pink elephant in your mind, and then try not to think about it. Remember: "try" is a presupposition to failure. It is impossible to not think about a pink elephant while you are thinking about a pink elephant. In addition, more emotional energy is attached to trying not to think about it than to think about it.

Let us explore how the law of reverse suggestion works for dieters. What you are saying in your mind is ***don't eat that chocolate ice cream***, which is really a hypnotic suggestion to "***eat that chocolate ice cream***!" The suggestibility to eat the ice cream then becomes stronger, and you use your willpower to say ***don't eat that chocolate ice cream!*** This is even worse because you have now linked the Law of Repetition to the Law of Reverse Suggestibility.

The force that you put into a reverse suggestion is returned to you with greater force. The harder you push the thought, the harder it is pushed back to you. The more times you push, the more times you are pushed. The stronger your willpower, the less effective it is. The more you will use repetition to give the counter-productive command of ***don't eat that chocolate ice cream***, the stronger the suggestion ***to eat that chocolate ice cream becomes***. The more you input this suggestion in your mind, the more powerfully it becomes imbedded in your imagination. *The ironic truth is: the stronger your willpower, the less likely you are to lose weight through the use of willpower.*

When I studied Judo, two of the first things that we were taught were the principles of tilting and kanting. When you kant, if you wish to throw a person forward, just prior to the throw, you give your opponent a quick, sharp push backward. Your opponent's natural reaction is to throw himself forward to keep from falling backwards. To illustrate how this reaction works for yourself, have someone apply resistance as you try to push their hand forward. Push so hard that they are having to push hard to keep you from pushing their hand backward, then quickly move your hand to the side and their hand will fly forward. This is a very good physical example of **the _psychological_** Law of Reverse Suggestion.

The judo player learns to push his opponent back quickly. His opponent begins to push forward quickly against the pressure, the judo player then pulls him forward, combining the power of his pull with the power of the opponent's push. Then the judo player uses his body to block the lower part of his opponent's body, thereby creating the very powerful throws of judo. A small man with technique can throw a big man. The bigger and stronger the opponent, the harder he or she falls. This is the literal truth behind the statement "The bigger they are, the harder that they fall."

If you put force behind a thought like ***"don't eat ice cream,"*** your mind will naturally resist that pressure. This is just the way the mind reacts. The more force that you apply, the greater the resistance.

You can think of it like this: the stronger you are, the bigger the snowball that you can roll uphill. The bigger the snowball, the more strength it derives from the principle of gravity. The Law of Reverse Suggestion operates like the principle of gravity. Gravity does not care whether or not you believe in it; gravity simply works on known principles. It is a power that can work against you and kill you if you step off a cliff without knowledge of the Law of Gravity. However, if you understand the principles upon which the Law of Gravity is based, you can harness and use its incredible power in the same way the power of a rushing river is converted to electrical energy. Once you understand the law, you never doubt that water flows downstream, and with this knowledge comes power.

If you understand that water flows downstream, but you desire to move water upstream, you can construct a simple waterwheel that is turned by the water rushing downstream. As it turns it tightens a rope attached to a pulley that carries a bucket of water to the top of the hill. In other words, you can learn to use the principle of gravity to your advantage by utilizing the power of gravity by altering the push of gravity and converting it to a pull.

Instead of saying, "Don't eat the chocolate ice cream," you should say, "Yes, there is chocolate ice cream and I will eat it if I *want* to." (This is changing the direction.) Then ask yourself, "Do I really want to eat the ice cream?" The question in itself creates doubt in the mind—a loss of faith in your *desire* to eat ice cream. To further weaken the suggestion, change the word "desire" to your passing thought of eating ice cream.

When you create that tiny space of doubt, follow it up with a barrage of questions like: is eating that fattening ice cream really more pleasurable than becoming slender, healthy, energetic, and sexy? Is eating a substance that is known to diminish the fires of my metabolism more pleasurable than drinking delicious, natural, healthy, body-purifying water?

If you come to the conclusion that eating the ice cream would be more pleasurable, tell yourself, "Okay, I will eat it, but I will only eat one bite at a time." Take a small bite, tasting the unhealthy substance upon the tip of your tongue, where the taste buds are the most sensitive. As you taste the fattening ice cream, really think about the taste. As you taste the ice cream, think about the negative consequences of eating it.

Once again, ask yourself if it really tastes *that good*. Give yourself a moment to reflect on whether it does or not. Go through this questioning process for two or three bites, and you will probably come to the conclusion that eating the ice cream just isn't worth it. Tell yourself that you would eat it if you *wanted* to, but you don't really *want* to. Now, while your old habit is on the ropes, throw in an affirmation like: "It is so much easier and more enjoyable to quench my thirst with a delicious glass of reverse osmosis water or spring water."

Press your advantage and ask yourself which is more delicious, purified water or natural spring water? Remember that the presupposition when you ask this question is that water is delicious. Ask yourself if you are going to have your water straight or with a touch of lemon in it. Will you be able to drink one or two glasses? Does water satisfy you because it is essential to all life or because you have suggested to yourself that it is satisfying?

In short, when you find yourself about to give yourself a negative reverse suggestion, turn it around by asking yourself questions that presuppose that you will eventually make a healthy choice because you *want* to make the healthy chose. The questions don't even have to make much sense. You could ask yourself, "Do I always make healthy choices because I am so good-looking, or is it because I am so darned smart?" The trick is to keep the focus away from using a reverse suggestion in a negative way.

This technique is much like a neuro-linguistic programming technique of interrupting the pattern. Every time your mind wanders to eating the chocolate ice cream, allow your mind to dream and drift to other unrelated subjects. Through practice, you can allow your mind to experience numerous humorous and distracting thoughts. Just don't practice the mental mind drifting technique when you are driving, operating heavy machinery, or when you should be attentive to your significant other. Failure to heed this warning could result in injury, death, or a nasty slap across the face.

Recognizing a reverse suggestion is 9/10 of the battle. Awareness is therapeutic in and of itself. With a sense of amusement, find how many times you catch yourself starting to give yourself a reverse suggestion. You may discover that this is an enjoyable game to play. With persistence you will all but eradicate your tendency to give yourself negative reverse suggestions.

17

The Law of Dominant Suggestion

If you have ever bought a cola at a movie theater, you have seen the Law of Dominant Suggestion in action. A very small cola, maybe a dime's worth, will sell for $2.50. A medium-size cola has twice as much cola, and it sells for $3.00. The large cola is twice as big as the medium cola, and it sells for $3.25. If you were any place but the movie theater, you would think that the price of cola is outrageously high. The strategy used in the movie theater is to establish the value of the cola via the inflated price of the small cola drink. Next to the small cola, the medium cola looks like a great value, and next to the medium cola, the large cola looks like a sensational deal. Using the Law of Dominant Suggestion, retailers have convinced you to buy more cola than you wanted or needed. They have also made you feel that you got a bargain.

If you wish to appear tall, take a picture of yourself standing beside someone who is very short. If you wish to appear to be a fast runner, run a race against someone who looks fast but is really slow. If you want to appear to be strong, lift something that looks heavy but is really very light.

If you want a suggestion to be very powerfully imbedded into your conscious and unconscious mind, pair it with a weaker suggestion. For example, if you want the phrase "nothing tastes as good as thin feels" to become a powerful thought in your mind, pair it with the phrase "every time I *think* of eating fattening foods I *know* that nothing tastes as good as thin feels." In this example, you have a weak suggestion ("think of eating fattening foods") paired with a stronger, or dominant, suggestion ("I know nothing tastes as good as thin feels"). Knowing is stronger than thinking, and by pairing a dominant suggestion with a weaker one, the suggestion becomes more powerful than when it is presented by itself.

Here is another example: whenever I *try* to eat something that is wrong for me, I *discover* that nothing tastes as good as thin feels. Discover is a stronger suggestion than try. Try is a presupposition to failure. Try to pick a pencil up from the table, and you will discover if you actually picked the pencil up from the table then you did not try. The word "try" does not exist unless you were unable to pick up the pencil. Try is an excellent weak suggestion that increases the power of corresponding dominant suggestions.

You could say, "Since I have started my hypnosis weight loss program, I find that the harder I *try* to overeat the harder it *becomes*. It is so much easier for me simply to allow myself to quit eating when I know that I am full." *To make any positive suggestion stronger, simply pair it with a weaker suggestion.* Note that the word allow is a presupposition that what you really *want* to do is to quit eating. "Try" leads one to the connotation that you really will not be able to overeat, and allow gives the connotation that what you really want to do is to quit eating when you are full.

Here is a list of words to put before a phrase to create a weak suggestion:

- Try
- Think,
- Hope
- Wish
- Believe
- Guess
- If
- May
- Might
- Could
- Like

Remember always to place one of these words in front of the suggestion that you want to be weak. For example, if you don't want to eat candy you might phrase a weak suggestion like this: "Even if I *wish* for a candy bar, I realize that I have no desire to eat one."

When you recognize that you have a thought to do something that does not support your weight loss goals, take a moment to figure out how to turn that thought into a weak suggestion followed by a dominant suggestion. By persistently practicing this technique, you will utilize three principles that have been presented in this book…

First, when you have the thought to eat a candy bar and you begin to think about changing it into a weak suggestion, you have to change the *focus* of your conscious mind from taking the action of eating the candy bar to taking the action of changing the thought of eating a candy bar to a weaker suggestion. Remember: *the conscious mind cannot think two separate thoughts at the same time.* As long as you are engaged in changing the suggestion to a weaker one, you will not be eating–provided you have accepted the suggestion not to eat anything without consciously thinking about it first.

Secondly, you convert the thought into a weaker suggestion. Without this conversion, the thought might have been "Wow, I am going to eat that candy bar right now." Instead, the suggestion is changed to something like "Whenever I have a *passing thought* of eating a candy bar, I smile with amusement and let it pass because I now *know* nothing tastes as good as thin feels."

Thirdly, you add a dominant suggestion, which is actually an affirmation to what would have been simply a command to eat something that would have made you fatter.

Take a few moments to verbalize some of the thoughts that have derailed you from losing weight in the past and figure out how to: (1) make those thoughts weak suggestions and (2) follow them with dominant suggestions. You can use the affirmations listed in this book as dominant suggestions; simply precede the appropriate affirmation with a word from the dominant suggestion list.

Here is a list of words to precede a dominant suggestion:

- Know
- Do
- Find
- Discover
- Realize
- When
- Will
- Would

When you practice this technique with persistence, you will discover that the dominant suggestions overpower the weaker suggestions, resulting in your changed behavior, and the ultimate weight loss that you desire. Notice that I have written this paragraph using words from the dominant list. Below I will re-write the paragraph using words from the weak suggestion list. Judge for yourself the power of each paragraph:

If you practice this technique with persistence, you may think that the dominant suggestion might overpower the weaker suggestion. Hopefully, it could change your behavior, and you may lose all the weight that you desire.

As weak as this suggestion is, this is the way most of us give ourselves positive suggestions. To prove my point: listen to your thought process sometime. Most of us state positive suggestions in this weak fashion. Have you ever said to yourself something like "I would like to lose a few pounds, but the older I am, the harder it gets"? Let us use the information that I have just given you to analyze this statement for a moment.

"I would *like* to lose a few pounds" is a very weak suggestion. This weak suggestion is followed by the dominant suggestion "The older I am, the harder it gets." Come on, I know that some of you are smiling with recognition because you have said something very similar to the statement that I just presented.

The tendency to make a positive suggestion weak and to follow it with a more dominant negative suggestion is so engrained that we don't even realize that we do it. I believe the reason why we have this tendency to give the positive suggestion to ourselves as a weak suggestion and then follow it with a strong or dominant suggestion is to protect ourselves from the disappointment of failure. Remember our basic need to avoid pain.

Most of us have been conditioned to believe that we should not get our *hopes* up too high. Notice even the thought of having our suggestions come true is weakened by the word "hope." Most of us are conditioned to believe that if you expect things to go well and they don't, it will hurt more than if you don't expect things to go well, and they still don't go well. This is common thinking for most of us, but *in reality this type of thinking is nothing more than a plan to fail!*

People have a tendency to cast doubt on anything that they have tried to do but failed. Because almost everybody in our society has tried to lose weight and failed, people have a tendency to give you the benefit of that experience. As general rule, people will indicate that your weight loss efforts will probably fail. The ironic thing is that *this thinking in and of itself is the real cause of failure in weight loss.*

In order to protect ourselves from the almost inevitable "it will not work" statement, we tend to phrase the statement weakly. Something like: "I am going to try to go on a diet again, but you know how that tends to go." When we use the word again, we are acknowledging that we have tried in the past and failed to lose weight. By acknowledging this up front, we know we take away some of the sting from being reminded that in the past we have tried and failed.

The next logical thing that anyone thinks is "In what way will this time be different from the last time?" People keep trying *new* diets and weight loss programs. We continue to have faith that the answer can be found in the *new* program or diet. The real answer cannot be found in the *new* diet or program. The real answer can only be found in the way we think about eating and exercise. If the new program causes us to think about eating and exercise differently it will work. However, when we try to plug a new diet into our existing patterns of thinking, we find that the new diet fails.

We gain *hope* (remember: hope is too weak; we need desire) of losing weight by having a new program in which to believe. We are able to elucidate intelligently the pros of this new diet or plan. We can recite the believable marketing spin that professional advertisers give to the new diet or program, but the truth is, *all diets work and all diets fail.*

Those people who learn to use desire, imagination, faith, and persistence in conjunction with the program or diet succeed, and those people who only use willpower or intellect ultimately fail. I am not casting stones. I am a professional hypnotist; I make my living using hypnosis to help people lose weight, and I know hypnosis works and I also know it doesn't work. It works for those people who learn the principles that I am teaching in this book, and it doesn't work for those people who fail to learn what I am teaching.

The whole message of this book is that weight loss must be preceded by a very powerful expectation that you will lose all the weight that you desire. This statement is the essential message of the chapter on faith. To be successful we must change our conditioning from doubt to faith. Faith is required to end our struggle with weight for life. We can change our conditions by learning how to give dominant suggestions to ourselves.

Below I will list a few poorly phrased suggestions that we frequently give ourselves when using the Law of Dominant Suggestion in exactly the opposite way than it should be applied. Then I will change the suggestion to one that better serves your interest.

Example # 1: I would like to lose weight, but everybody in my family is overweight.

Analysis # 1: Like is a weak suggestion and it is followed by the idea that I have a genetic condition that will prevent me from losing weight.

Correction # 1: When I use these principles to lose all the weight that I desire, I will be able to teach other members of my family to lose weight.

Analysis of correction # 1: The word "when" presupposes that it will happen. The phrase "I will teach other members of my family to do it" negates the possibility that genetics will keep you from losing weight.

Example # 2: No matter how hard I try, I can't seem to lose weight. I guess my willpower is too weak.

Analysis of #2: Try is a presupposition to failure. The use of "hard" indicates it will be painful and "my willpower is too weak" is a statement expressing that I just don't have the innate ability to lose weight.

Correction of example # 2: I will lose all the weight that I desire because this time I am not using my willpower; I am using the power of my imagination. I know that whenever imagination and willpower come into conflict, imagination *always* wins!

Analysis of correction for example # 2: The use of will indicates a positive statement. Next, a logic rationale for why this time will be different is indicated, and the last statement, "imagination always wins," is an affirmation and a presupposition that you *will* win and lose all the weight that you desire to lose.

Example # 3: I know that I could lose weight if it wasn't for my thyroid problem.

Analysis for example #3: Although "know" is a power word, the power is reversed to weakness when it is followed by the word "could." The stronger suggestion is that the thyroid problem will keep you from losing all the weight that you desire.

Correction for example #3: I will feel much more healthy and energetic when I lose all the weight that I desire to lose.

Analysis of correction # 3: This is just a strong statement using the words "will" and "desire" and the statement presupposes that you will lose all the weight that you desire. It is better not to mention the thyroid. You may actually have a thyroid problem, but dwelling on that problem will be counterproductive to your efforts to lose weight.

Therefore, allow the passing thought of your thyroid to float from your mind and die from lack of attention.

Mastering the concept of the Law of Dominate Suggestion is easy to do. When you have mastered this law you will be well on your way to ending the struggle with weight management for life.

18

The Power of Emotions

A thought is like a bullet. If placed in the right gun, aimed correctly, and fired with enough velocity; it will hit its target. Most of this book has been about using your gun (your mind), making your own bullets (thoughts), aiming them correctly (your goals), and firing them enough times (repetition) to kill the beast (habits that lead to being overweight). This chapter is all about the ingredient that gives your bullets velocity and knock down power.

Emotions are the gunpowder of this process. The overweight habit beast can be a huge, tough, and resilient animal. In our country, 65 percent of the people who fight against this animal, lose. This is not surprising since most of the people in this country really don't understand how their gun works. They don't practice aiming their gun, and they really don't even have a target. They use bullets made by someone who does not want them to kill the beast, and they don't use the gunpowder that is available to them. Just think about this analogy for a minute, or two, and compare it with what I write next.

If you are reading or listening to this book you definitely have a mind, but prior to reading this book you might not have understood how the mind actually works. It is as if you have this incredible gun, but you don't have an owner's manual. You really have little understanding of how the weapon operates. This is understandable for we receive no formal training in how our minds actually work.

I believe that someday the principles that I am sharing with you will be among the very first subjects that we teach children when they begin school. People are beginning to discover the scientific principles of thinking. Today that science is hypnosis. Hypnosis is an unfortunate name because the name is steeped in cultural mythology, and most people's knowledge of hypnosis is inaccurate. To coin a phrase, I prefer to call the body of principles that explain the phenomenon of hypnosis as the "Science of Suggestion."

The important thing to note is, there now exists a body of scientific principles that reveal the secrets of the mind. Hypnosis and neural-linguistic programming are leading the way in developing this new science. As Shakespeare said, "A rose by any other name would still smell as sweet." For now, let us simply say this book is about is the science of suggestibility as it specifically applies to weight loss and weight management.

Numerous times I have said that we have the power to control our thoughts. However, for the most part, we do not create our own thoughts. We mistakenly believe that it is so much easier to accept thoughts proffered by television, radio, newspapers, friends, relatives, and even enemies than it is to develop our own thoughts.

The truth is, ultimately it is much easier for us to control our own thoughts than to deal with the endless problems that occur when we allow others to choose our thoughts for us. I challenge you to grasp what I am saying and practice the principles taught in this book. I challenge you *to take control of your own thoughts and to create your own destiny.*

For the moment, concentrate on controlling your thoughts about eating and exercise. You will know from the changing shape of your body and from your increasing vigor, energy, and enjoyment of life that these principles work. You will have proof positive which will instill faith in you, then you will be able to apply this same thinking process to every other area of your life.

Now back to the business of losing weight. You have been learning how your mind works and how to control the direction of your thoughts; now you must learn how to put plenty of power behind the thoughts. As we have discussed, our eating is unconscious, and changing the conditioned responses of the unconscious mind is the only way to end the battle with weight problems. *Emotions are the language that the unconscious mind understands.*

As we have discussed, hypnosis, autosuggestion, and the repetition of affirmations are capable of penetrating our critical filters and entering into the realm of the unconscious mind. We must first enter the realm of the unconscious mind in order to change the conditioned response or habit. This chapter is about giving you another technique to change habits. This technique can be used separately or in combination with hypnosis, affirmations, and autosuggestion. The secret to the technique is this: *Any suggestion paired with strong emotion has the power to stop the critical filter and immediately change the conditioned response. If the emotion is strong enough, the change can be permanently accomplished in one time.*

Let me give you an example of how this could occur. Let us assume that a lady walks to her car in a dark parking lot. She gets into the car, and a man in the back of the car puts a knife to her throat. Immediately, she knows that her life is threatened, and she feels fear.

Fear triggers her "flight or fight" mechanism. Her body prepares to fight or to run. The heart begins beating faster, pumping oxygen to the blood. The breath comes in quick gasps, again sending the oxygen to the muscles. Adrenalin is pumped throughout her body. The skin becomes whiter as blood rushes from the face so that if she gets cut, she won't bleed as badly. Her body is preparing to run faster or fight more powerfully than ever before. In a fight, instead of thinking consciously, she will react automatically, because the critical filter has been short-circuited and unconscious mind has taken control. This process releases an automatic response that has allowed our species to survive.

Very powerful emotions like fear trigger this fight or flight response. Other emotions will be triggered as well. In that moment, she may feel that she is going to die. She may think of her small child growing up without a mother, thereby triggering the emotion of love for her child. She may think of this stranger depriving her child of a mother; thus the emotion of anger is triggered. She decides to fight. Driven by these powerful emotions, she fights with great strength and speed. She frees herself from the assailant, nimbly gets out of the car, and runs like the wind to safety.

The entire episode took less than six seconds, and yet from now on she will be afraid to get into a car in a dark parking lot. We can say that she has been traumatized, but what has really happened, is the strong emotions short-circuited her critical filter, and in a heartbeat a new habit was established. The habit of getting into her car without fear was replaced by the new habit of being fearful of getting into the car. Notice that no progressive relaxation was used. There was no affirmation or autosuggestion, and in one fleeting instance the habit was radically changed. The stronger the emotions are, the quicker and more dramatic the change.

Now that we understand how this lightning-fast change of neural-associations can take place, how do we use this information to facilitate our weight loss? Do you really think that I would suggest that you hire someone to hold a knife to your throat every time you try to eat something that is bad for you? Well–not exactly, but you could allow the emotion of fear to become a counselor to you. Let me explain how this technique could work for you.

Quoting Weight Loss International: "Being overweight has profound health implications. Obesity significantly increases a person's risk of a number of life-threatening conditions, such as diabetes, heart disease, stroke, high blood pressure, and some types of cancer, according to recent obesity in America statistics." Being overweight has recently surpassed smoking to become the most reliable predictor of a shorter life span. We even have a term known as "morbidly obese." If you are obese or if you have been gaining 5 or 10 or more pounds a year at that rate, it will not be long before you will be morbidly obese. In reality, your life is in danger. You are literally killing yourself with your glutinous habits.

The chances are that just by being overweight, you will prematurely deprive the people you love of your presence in this life. Picture those people who are dear to you, and feel the grief that they will experience when you eat your self to death. Make the pictures in your imagination very vivid because *the imagination has no ability to distinguish what is real and what is fantasy.* If you make the pictures real in your imagination, they will become real. The mind tends to produce what is *persistently* held in the imagination. The key word here is "persistently."

In order to create some powerful emotion, try this exercise: see yourself eating fattening food, gorging yourself, killing yourself with your glutinous habits. See the pain on the faces of your loved ones as they try to stop you while you continue to eat, and then imagine yourself incredibly fat and bloated in a coffin. Associate the pain of this experience with the fattening foods that you once thought that you enjoyed. Realize that you essentially poisoned yourself to death and died for nothing.

You failed to accomplish your mission in life because of your indulgences. Allow yourself to become angry with yourself. Associate these miserable feelings with those fattening foods until the very sight of those foods disgusts you.

There is no doubt that this is a very morbid and painful exercise, but at this point it is only in your imagination. Just briefly create the experiences in your imagination until you feel strong emotions, and then let this negative picture disappear.

Never do this negative exercise without following it with a positive one! Now imagine yourself as healthy, lean, fit, and attractive. See yourself as self-confident, brimming with energy, and experiencing a very strong sense of serenity. This is the picture that you want to hold persistently in your imagination.

Use the driving force of sex to powerfully imprint a desired behavior. When it comes to the desire to gain pleasure, sex is the most powerful of all emotions. There is a natural link between having a lean, healthy, sexy body and enjoying sexual pleasure. Use this natural link to associate sexual pleasure with your new eating and exercise habits.

Instead of fantasizing about eating something unhealthy, allow yourself to remember or fantasize enjoying a sexual experience with your significant other. Then pair this feeling to a desire to eat healthy foods or to do an exercise that you want to enjoy.

If you do not have a sexual relationship with anyone at the moment, think of someone with whom you would like to have a relationship, and use this motivation to drive yourself to become leaner and sexier.

I am not here to preach any type of religious doctrine. My goal is to give you a very simple and practical handbook for changing your thinking so that you can achieve your weight-loss goal. This book is about growing new thoughts in the garden of your mind. It is my belief that the more you can free yourself of negative feelings like jealousy, anger, anxiety, fear, resentment, etc., the more fertile the soil of your mind becomes.

While it is true that negative emotions such as fear, anger, and revenge can be very powerful motivators when harnessed and channeled to a definite major purpose, it is my belief that you will be a happier and healthier person by harnessing the power of positive emotions instead. Fear should be a counselor to you. The need to avoid pain can motivate you to improve. However, when you have built your plan, and are walking confidently in the direction of your goal, your fear should disperse.

If you have a very powerful negative emotion (or emotions) with which you are dealing, you should allow yourself to let go of it. Most religious organizations can get you in touch with people who can help you learn love, forgiveness, and peace. Most spiritual practices will teach you techniques to let go of negative feelings and emotions to become more peaceful. Psychologists and hypnotists can help you to release negative feelings.

Negative feelings give rise to negative emotions and thoughts, and unhappy negative thoughts tend to cloak themselves in the misery of excess fat. Release the resentment or anger that you hold for another person, and you may discover that you release the excess weight as well. Letting go of your guilt can allow you to let go of your extra pounds.

19

Exercise Motivation

In this chapter you will learn three components of exercising motivation: (1) End Results Imagery, (2) Immediate State Change, and (3) Under Promise and Over Deliver.

I have talked a great deal about end results imagery. Basically this technique is linking massive amounts of pleasure with becoming your ideal weight and size. Remember that humans are mainly motivated by just two things: (1) the need to avoid pain and (2) the desire to gain pleasure.

What happens when the human mind is confronted with pain and pleasure in conflict? For example, you may feel pain because you are flabby, out of shape, and not as attractive as you could be. Therefore you go to the gym to work out, yet when you get there you begin to experience the pain of your workout. You have the pain of working out vs. the pain of being out of shape. You are motivated to avoid pain, so which do you choose?

You will choose the pain that is most real to you at that moment. If you have a burning desire to be in shape, you will have to make that desire more real than the pain of working out. As a hypnotist I was taught that 20 percent of pain is experienced locally, and 80 percent is experienced in the mind. It is interesting to note that *the expectation of pain is more painful than the pain itself.* I know that sounds crazy, but it really is true.

There have been experiments where people were brought to a dentist with the expectation that the procedure would be very painful. The dentist revved up his drills to make noise and then lightly touched the patient with a soft spongy instrument. The patient then experienced intense levels of pain. Conversely, there have been very painful dental procedures in which the dentist has reassured the patient that there will be little pain, and the patient then experienced a minimal amount of pain.

Many dentists and other doctors use hypnosis effectively to control pain. Hypnosis is used thousands of times each year to assist mothers in making childbirth a vastly less painful experience. Soldiers and professional athletes have conditioned their minds to tolerate what most of us would consider intolerable amounts of pain and still perform at peak levels with a minimum amount of discomfort.

You can condition yourself to think of your workout as vastly more enjoyable than it is painful. You can even link the 20 percent actual pain with becoming more fit, healthy, and attractive and thereby begin to form a pleasurable association.

Arnold Schwarzenegger was reported as saying a good muscle pump was better than sex. I don't quite claim *that* (a man has to draw the line somewhere), but because the perception of pleasure is created in the mind, it is possible to condition yourself to believe this way.

This conditioning can be done through the use of hypnosis, autosuggestion, affirmations, and the power of emotion. In the back of the book, I have created a hypnosis script for exercise motivation; the suggestions in the script can also be used as affirmations and autosuggestions.

When you reach this pain vs. pain conflict of two opposing pains (for example: (1) the pain of working out and (2) the pain of being flabby and out of shape), both pains appear to be equally real. So which one do you choose? *You will choose to avoid the pain or gain the pleasure that seems to be more immediate!*

This statement means that it is helpful to link *immediate* pleasure with working out. You can condition yourself to experience the pleasure of a slightly elevated heart beat, the way it feels when your muscles move smoothly and fluidly, the feel of a light glistening sweat, the tight firm feeling of a muscle when it is gorged, or the pleasant feeling of breathing deeply after exertion.

The trick is to enjoy and savor these sensations as pleasurable. What do you do if these sensations don't seem to feel pleasurable to you? You simply pretend that they are pleasurable until they actually become pleasurable. If you are persistent in pretending, you will convince yourself.

Whatever experience you wish to become stronger in your life should be linked to a real and immediate pleasure. How real and immediate that sensation is, is subject to your control, for *you have the power to control your thoughts!*

The third principle of exercise motivation is Under Promise and Over Deliver. I also refer to this as my 70 percent principle. *Nothing motivates like success.* The successful completion of a long or short-term goal is registered in the mind as a success. Therefore *when you exercise, you always want to set yourself up to be successful.*

It is important to note that the psychology of aerobic and strength training exercise is very different. Some of the advantages of aerobic training are improving your physical fitness, strengthening your heart, and burning massive amounts of calories. Strength training will build lean muscle mass, increase your strength, and give your body that sexy athletic look. The lean muscle mass will speed up your metabolism, causing your body to burn more calories even when you are at rest. Ideally, you will incorporate both types of exercise into your weight-loss program. However, you will need a different mindset for strength training than you do for aerobic training.

Here is how the 70 percent principle works with regard to strength training. If you absolutely know that you can do 10 repetitions of an exercise with maximum exertion, then tell yourself that you need to do seven (70 percent) to be successful. If you do seven, you will be successful. As you start to do the repetitions, tell yourself that when you do four you will be over halfway to your goal.

When you reach four, realize that effort wasn't so hard, and go for your goal of seven. As you do seven, say to yourself that you still feel strong and that it would be a fun challenge to see how many repetitions beyond seven you can do. If you reach nine, feel proud of yourself for having exceeded your goal by two, and challenge yourself to exceed it by even more next time. You feel good because not only have you achieved your goal, you have overachieved, and you overachieved not because you had to, but because you *wanted* to. Now you begin to think of wanting to exercise instead of having to exercise.

Compare this way of thinking with the way people usually think: "I have to reach 10 to be successful." "I don't feel very good today, and I doubt I will be able to do 10." "Oh no, I am on one. That is a [expletive deleted] long way from 10." "Four? Oh man, I am not even halfway there." "Seven? Oh shoot me, three more to go. I will never make it!" "Nine. That is it; I can't do another one." "I knew I didn't feel good." "I must be doing something wrong; I keep working out but I never get any stronger." "Why do I even bother?"

Always set yourself up to be successful. When you are successful, you begin to think of yourself as an overachiever, and you begin to expect success. You will develop pride. You will realize that you are a person of volition and that whatever you set out to accomplish will be accomplished and that is a fact as irrefutable as your ability to read the words on this page.

When you are involved in an aerobic training exercise like jogging, the psychology is different. An interesting thing about aerobic exercise is that the first five minutes are the most difficult. People who set a goal to jog for 15 minutes or more usually fail within the first five minutes. After five minutes, jogging becomes easier. You begin to catch your second wind. Your body loosens up, and you begin to move more fluidly and easily. Therefore, when you begin to run, focus on making the first five minutes. Tell yourself that after five minutes, it gets easier.

Focus on your breathing; the rhythm and fluidity of your movements. Choose an affirmation from the back of the book or write your own. Repeat the affirmation (out loud or in your mind). The idea is to distract your mind. Allow this running behavior to become an unconscious behavior for a time.

The rewards of exercise are so tremendous that you will become addicted to it. Think of yourself as a healthy, strong, fit, and attractive person. Begin to train for recreational activities that you find enjoyable. Whether you choose to hike, swim, play tennis, climb mountains, ride bikes, etc., is not important as long as you experience real enjoyment in that activity. Becoming a well-conditioned person will add a whole new dimension of pleasure to your life.

20

Helping Others to Lose Weight

My father had a favorite joke about five boy scouts who were assigned to do a good deed in order to earn their merit badges. Each of the five boys reported that they had helped a little old lady go across the street. The scoutmaster said, "You mean all of you helped little old ladies across the street?" The boys replied, "Not little old ladies; just one little old lady." The scoutmaster inquired, "You mean it took all five of you to help one little old lady to cross the street?" The boys responded, "Yes, sir. She didn't want to go."

This joke is my way of saying never offer to help someone to lose weight. The best way to help others is to be a role model and lose weight yourself. Invariably, when you become your ideal weight and size, people will begin to ask you how you did it. I place these people in two categories: (1) those who are just curious and (2) those who are seriously seeking to lose weight and become healthier.

In my personal experience, nothing is more gratifying and fulfilling than to teach another person how to utilize the principles presented in this book to lose all of the weight that they desire to lose. I can also tell you that nothing is more futile than to attempt to help someone who is not committed to losing weight. The desire and commitment must begin in each and every person. Unfortunately, the battle of the bulge is a battle that must be fought by one soldier at a time.

If you decide to help someone to lose weight, it is important not to argue with them about the specifics of losing weight. Most people feel like they already know what they need to do. In my experience, there is simply no specific pat formula for losing weight.

There are, however, four simple principles that, when mastered, assure weight loss.

Simply focus on helping your friend to: (1) create a burning desire to lose weight, (2) actively use his or her imagination to lose weight, (3) develop the faith and self-confidence that he or she needs to lose all the desired weight, and (4) enjoy some type of exercise. If you will simply focus on these four things, you will not only have helped your friend, you will have strengthened your relationship with your friend.

Everybody needs a coach, a friend, and a cheerleader. Nothing is more gratifying than to serve in these capacities and to watch your friends achieve their goals.

I wish you the best of good fortune in achieving your personal goals and helping others to achieve theirs.

21

Weight Loss Affirmations

Affirmations play a very important role in your weight loss program for the following two reasons: (1) repetition is the mother of learning and (2) you can use affirmations to change the focus of your mind from negative, fearful thoughts of doubt to powerful, positive thoughts of faith.

You simply cannot imprint a positive thought into your mind too many times. When you pair an affirmation with a positive emotion of love, faith, friendship, sex, or compassion, it *becomes your thought.*

You can become a positive, optimistic, determined, and successful person by imprinting positive thoughts into your unconscious mind. No matter where you are or what is happening, you can always choose a positive affirmation to say silently in your mind. At times, you will also be able to say the affirmation out loud with strength and conviction. *You can never repeat a good affirmation too many times.*

Affirmations can be used to protect you from the many negative or fearful thoughts that will come to you unbidden. You can always choose to counter a negative thought with a corresponding positive affirmation. You can do this instantly, anytime, anywhere.

Your mind is thinking thoughts continually, and the thoughts you think manifest into what we know as reality. Therefore, *think thoughts about what you do want, not about what you don't want.* The concept is so simple and yet so powerful. The mastery of this one technique alone can reprogram your mind so that losing weight and maintaining that weight loss becomes as automatic as breathing. You can choose your own reality by learning to practice persistently these simple principles of affirmation.

There is no real secret to affirmations as long as they are positive and directly support your definite major goals. I have listed many affirmations with regard to weight loss. You may choose from the list below or develop your own, but it is a good idea to have a few affirmations memorized to defend yourself against the negative thoughts that will encroach into the territory of your mind.

- Nothing tastes as good as thin feels.

- I enjoy eating healthy and nutritious foods in just the right amount.

- I know when I have eaten just the right amount; it is when I reach that point I become completely satisfied.

- I enjoy drinking delicious water and I find it is becoming my beverage of choice, both at meals and in between meals.

- I enjoy my weight loss program; food is becoming less and less important to me.

- I know that the pleasure of eating comes from the taste, texture, and flavor of the food, and these are all things that I can enjoy better when I eat more slowly.

- I can experience more pleasure by eating less.

- Whenever I eat smaller portions at night, I find that when my head hits the pillow, I drift into a dreamy sleep, sleeping quickly, deeply, and soundly, sleeping throughout the night, dreaming beautiful dreams, and awakening refreshed, energized, and highly motivated to continue my weight loss program.

- I eat my food slowly, savoring each and every bite, and because I eat slowly I realize when I have reached that place of perfect nutritional comfort–and I find I lose the desire to eat past that point of satisfaction and comfort.

- Whenever I think of eating, I think of healthy nutritious food.

- I find that I am losing the wish to eat foods that are bad for me.

- If I try to eat something that is bad for me, I find after a bite or two that food tastes disgusting.

- The harder I try to eat fattening foods the harder it is. It is just so much easier to allow myself to drink delicious water.

- Whenever I drink water, I am more energized.

- I find myself wanting to exercise at every possible opportunity.

- I enjoy exercising more and more each and every day.

- I look forward to exercising.

- I enjoy the pleasant feeling of soreness in my muscles.

- As I exercise, I can feel my fat melting away.

- When I walk, each and every step brings me closer to my goal of losing all the weight that I desire.

- After I exercise, I walk tall, straight, and proud.

- As I exercise, I can feel my muscles growing bigger, stronger, harder, and leaner.

- It is fun to exercise.

- As I exercise, I can feel myself becoming a more powerful, purposeful, and attractive person.

- Because I exercise I look good in whatever clothes I wear. I would rather have a good body and be wearing jeans than have a fat body in expensive clothes.

- As I exercise my muscles, I also exercise my character.

- When I set an exercise goal, I get a great deal of pleasure from achieving that goal.

- Losing weight is a fun and stimulating game that I enjoy playing and winning.

- Nothing tastes as good as it feels to be fit, firm, and in great shape.

- Because I exercise regularly, my biological age is years younger than my chronological age.

- When I exercise and eat right, I move lightly with fluid grace and agility.

- Exercising regularly is a gift that I give myself.

- I would rather use my gym membership than use my medical insurance.

- Because I exercise I am confident that I can protect myself.

- Because I exercise regularly now, as I get older I am better conditioned and more attractive.

- My sex life is great because I enjoy exercising.

- When I exercise, my stresses just seem to disappear.

- I love how I feel after a good sweat.

- I enjoy challenging my muscles by lifting weights.

- Nothing feels as good as a good muscle pump.

- I am becoming stronger every day in each and every way!

22

Self Hypnosis Induction Scripts and Weight Loss Suggestions

Before you read the hypnosis scripts that follow, you should know that hypnosis is not a magical or mystical experience, and *yet it is very powerful*. Hypnosis is in fact a naturally occurring phenomenon. You are in a state of deep hypnosis at least twice a day. Each night when you go from a waking state to sleep or from beta to delta you go through alpha (light hypnosis) and theta (deep hypnosis) to delta (deep sleep).

Under hypnosis there will never be a time when you will be in a trance so deep that you cannot awaken from it. You will always hear and be aware of everything going on. At no time will you surrender your will. You will always be in charge of you. As a matter of fact, since you have consciously chosen the suggestions that you will give to yourself, self-hypnosis is a time when you are more in charge of your thinking process than ever before.

Hypnosis is like anything else: the more you practice, the better you become. There is really no way to mess up the hypnotic experience. If you feel even a mild level of relaxation, the experience has been successful and worthwhile. As you practice, the experience will become even stronger.

Many of you will experience a very profound sense of relaxation from the very first time you practice. For many of you, the result will be instant and truly amazing. Others will need to practice to achieve the remarkable results that are imminently possible. It is my most fervent belief that that self-hypnosis will work for anyone of reasonable intelligence, imagination, motivation, and persistence.

Simply read the scripts that follow; choose your favorite induction script; record it, and follow it with the therapeutic suggestions listed at the end of this chapter. If you prefer, you can simply order the appropriate CD from me. Order forms are included in the back of the book.

The Basic Induction

Hypnosis is created using words,
words can make us angry,
words can make us sad,
the use of words
can create anxiety
or evoke deep feelings
of relaxation and
serenity
words can also evoke feelings
of physical sensations
in the body
feelings of lightness
or heaviness
feelings of hot or cold
as you go through the process,
of hypnosis
a number of thoughts and images
may come to mind,
thoughts of whether or not
you are really being hypnotized,
whenever you have the thought of
whether or not you are really
being hypnotized,
just pretend that you really are
being hypnotized,
and as you are pretending that
you are really being hypnotized,
simply pretend that you are
not pretending,
you really are being hypnotized,
and the mind
and the body
just begins to relax
a little more than before,
as you allow yourself
to become more

peaceful
more and more relaxed
than before,
and you can allow that alteration
to occur,
and you can drift away on words,
whenever you get the chance,
and chances are
you will become more relaxed, and
more peaceful
than you have ever known yourself
to be,
during the process of hypnosis,
you may begin to experience
a number of physiological
reactions taking place
in the body,
in a few moments,
you may begin to realize
that your attention is drawn
toward your breathing,
when you first begin
to realize
that your attention is drawn toward
your breathing,
simply nod your head yes,
as you nod your head yes,
the mind and body
begin to experience
the gentle drifting
as it occurs
for you have known
all along that
as the body relaxes
the mind relaxes as well,
and you can feel yourself
breathing
more deeply

more rhythmically than before,
and you can allow yourself
to experience that gentle
letting go,
in a few moments,
you may begin
to experience
a dryness in your lips,
your lips may begin to feel
very dry and parched
as if you had been out
in the hot, hot sun
and the wind
for a very long time,
and this feeling of dryness
in the lips
may become
so profound that
you may experience
a desire to just want to
lick your lips,
when you first begin
to notice that you have
a tendency to
just want to lick
your lips,
simply nod your head yes
and as you nod your head yes
this feeling of relaxation continues
to deepen
a little more
than before,
and the mind and the body
continue to relax,
as you breathe deeply,
breathing in relaxation,
and breathing out tension,
inhaling relaxation, and

exhaling tension
with each and every word
that you hear,
and you *can drift* away on words,
in a few moments,
you may begin to experience
an accumulation of
saliva
in your mouth,
you can realize that
the saliva accumulates more
with each and every word that
you hear,
with each and every breath that
you take,
this accumulation
of saliva
may become
so pronounced and
so profound that
you have a desire to
just want to
swallow,
when you first begin
to notice
that you do have a desire to
just want to
swallow,
simply
nod your head yes,
that's right,
and the mind
and the body
continues to relax
more and more
than before,
as you allow yourself to
dream, drift and drop,

and it feels so good to
enjoy this feeling of
letting go,
and you can experience
a very pleasant
tingling sensation occurring
in the top
of your scalp,
and you can feel
this pleasant tingling sensation
as it begins to flow
into your forehead,
just smoothing out all
the tiny little lines
on the forehead
with relaxation,
as this wonderful
tingling sensation
begins to relax
all the muscles of the
the face,
and the area between your
mouth and your ears
may experience such
profound relaxation
that your mouth may
want to part slightly
in relaxation, and
if it does,
that is fine,
because it all belongs
to you,
and all the tensions
and stresses of the day
just seem to want to
go to and accumulate
in the neck,
but you can feel this

pleasant tingling sensation
of relaxation
just chasing all the tensions
and stresses
of the day
away
and you can allow yourself to
dream, drift, and drop,
as you go down to a very
pleasant place of
comfort and relaxation,
and the tingling relaxing feeling
continues to spread,
moving from the neck
to the shoulders,
you can experience that
relaxation in the shoulders
as it occurs,
and begins to move gently
into the arms,
relaxing the biceps
and the triceps,
and just sliding down to
lubricate and relax the elbow,
as the elbow becomes
loose, limp, and relaxed,
the relaxing sensation
just begins to flow into
the forearms,
slowly spreads to the wrists,
as you experience this feeling
of relaxation
in the palms
of your hands,
and as you do
it quickly spreads to
each and every finger,
and to the thumbs as well,

the white light shines on
your chest
and as it does
you can feel your chest relax,
as this sensation curves around to
your back,
just relaxing each and every
major and minor muscle
in the back,
now wonderful feeling
begins to just
gravitate toward and
slide down your
spinal column,
relaxing each and every vertebra
on the way down,
down past the middle back,
down to the lower back,
and spreading to relax
all the muscles of the
lower back,
as this sensation of
relaxation
curves around your stomach,
relaxing all the muscles in
the stomach,
and now the
stomach, chest, and back
are relaxed,
and all the internal organs inside
just begin to slow down with
relaxation,
your heartbeat
begins to slow down
with relaxation,
flowing down
with relaxation
into your lap, and

the mind and the body
began to relax even more,
and more than before,
with each and every breath
that you take
you feel this profound
feeling of spreading relaxation,
as it moves to your hips,
you feel the spreading
relaxation
in your hips, and
it just begins
to flow into your legs,
relaxing your inner thighs,
and your outer thighs,
and you can experience
that tingly relaxing feeling,
as it lubricates your knees,
with a pleasant relaxing feeling,
that wonderful feeling just begins
to slip down,
down into your
shins and calves,
just sliding down,
down into your ankles,
leaving them
loose, limp, and relaxed,
as you experience
that sensation of relaxation
in your feet
it quickly begins to spread
to each and every toe
on your feet,
and now you are relaxed
from the tip
of your toes
to the top
of your scalp,

and as the body relaxes,
the mind relaxes as well,
relaxes with it,
and into it,
for you have known all along,
that you learn better when
you are relaxed,
and now you are in a very
powerful place of learning,
you are free to
accept the suggestions
that I give to you now
into the most powerful part
of your unconscious mind,
and these suggestions
will become a part
of your automatic thinking,
they will become as automatic
as your breathing...
Note: The basic induction has concluded. Please insert the suggestions listed at the end of this chapter.

Magical Forest Induction

In order to become
even more relaxed
than before,
I want you to imagine yourself
in a wonderfully magical rain forest,
night has just fallen, and
it is a beautiful indigo blue night,
the stars are shining and glittering, in
a vast display of beauty,
they fill the night sky
like sparkling diamonds on
a black velvet cloak,
as you look into this amazing night sky,
you see the biggest most beautiful moon, that
you have ever seen in your life,
a full moon,
a harvest orange moon,
so big and bright that
you can see the mountains on
that moon with the naked eye,
and as you glance up at this amazing moon,
you begin to notice,
a white light emanating from it,
as you look up,
this light begins
to shine down
on you,
just touching the tip of your scalp,
and as it does
it leaves your scalp with a
pleasant tingly sensation of
relaxation, peace, and serenity,
this wonderful feeling of relaxation,
begins to flow down to
your forehead,
just smoothing all the tiny little lines

with relaxation,
the white light baths your face,
and your entire face begins to relax,
the muscles in your cheeks relax,
your nose relaxes,
your lips and chin begin to relax,
and the area between the mouth and
the ears may begin to experience such
a profound sense of relaxation
that your jaw may become so relaxed
that your mouth just wants to part
slightly in relaxation,
and if it does
that is fine
because it all belongs to you,
all the tensions and stresses
of the day just seem to want to
go to and accumulate in the neck,
but the white light touches the neck,
and all the tensions and stresses are
simply chased away,
and the mind and the body,
begin to relax more and more
than before,
this pleasant tingly sensation of relaxation,
goes down
and flows down
to the shoulders,
and as it relaxes
the shoulders
this wonderful sensation of relaxation,
quickly flows into the arms,
relaxing the biceps and triceps,
as it flows down to the elbows,
leaving the elbows feeling
lubricated and relaxed,
and the feeling continues to flow
into the forearms,

relaxing each and every muscle
of the forearm,
and moving into the wrist
leaving the wrist very loose, limp and relaxed,
you may begin to experience this sensation
of relaxation,
in the palm of the hands
and as you do
it quickly spreads to
each and every finger
on your hands and to
the thumbs as well,
the white light just touches your chest,
and your chest begins to experience that relaxation,
as the white light curves to your back,
relaxing all the major muscles of the back,
and just sliding down the spinal column,
relaxing each and every vertebra
as it slides down, down, down,
to the lower back,
with relaxation flowing outward
to relax all the major and minor muscles
of the lower back,
then curving around to the stomach,
now the stomach, chest, and back
are relaxed,
and as they relax,
all the internal organs inside,
just begin to relax as well,
the white light shines on your lap,
and the lap begins to enjoy that
feeling of relaxation,
as it spreads
to the hips,
relaxing both hips,
and moving
to the legs
as it moves through the legs,

relaxing the inner thighs,
and the outer thighs,
just sliding down,
to lubricate and relax
the knee joints,
as your experience this wonderful feeling
of relaxation in the knees,
it just begins to slip to the shins,
as it curves around to the calves,
now slipping to the ankles,
and the ankles become
very loose, limp, and relaxed,
you can experience that
tingly sensation in the feet,
as it spreads quickly
to each and every
toe on the feet,
and now your body
is relaxed
from the tip of your toes,
to the top of your scalp,
as the body relaxes,
the mind relaxes as well,
relaxes with it, into it,
as you allow yourself to
dream, drift, and drop,
to dream away for a time,
allowing yourself to go
deeper, and deeper,
into a place of deep serenity,
allowing yourself to become
more peaceful than you have ever known
yourself to be,
and the mind and the body relax,
more and more than before,
in order to become even
more relaxed
I want you to imagine

a magnificent tree
a tree so tall,
that the top of the tree
is lost in the clouds,
a tree trunk so large
that it extends beyond your field of vision,
the tree trunk is hollow,
and in the middle of a great hollow tree,
there is a beautiful oak door,
and as you approach the oak tree,
you see a sign above the tree,
saying "Now Showing:
[YOUR FAVORITE MOVIE]"
you can feel yourself gripping
the polished brass doorknob,
you can feel the slight pull
of the door as
it smoothly opens up,
revealing a very spacious
beautiful and magical movie theater,
you stand in darkness for one brief moment,
as your eyes accustom themselves
to the darkness,
you begin to see with clarity,
in that beautiful,
but dimly lit movie theater,
the usher politely
shows you to
the most comfortable chair
that you could possibly imagine,
you wait for only a moment,
and the movie begins,
you see a very slender and attractive person,
on the movie screen,
this person is walking through
a verdant and pristine rain forest,
you notice how lightly she walks,
she moves with effortless ease,

gliding with agility, grace,
self-confidence, and poise,
exuding energy, vitality, health,
and a zestful passion for life,
as the camera comes in for a close-up,
that person smiles into the camera,
you find with a sense of wonderment,
that you on the movie screen,
the ideal you,
your perfect weight and size,
you notice the smallness of your waist,
you notice your firm, toned legs, hips, and arms,
you find with a sense of pride,
that you have become your ideal weight and size,
you know you are seeing the real you,
the you inside of you,
you notice the people around you
at the theater,
the chairs are filled with your family,
friends, and co-workers,
you see the look of respect and admiration
on their faces,
as they watch you on the movie screen,
you are proud to know that
you have achieved your weight loss goals,
simply by allowing the suggestions
that I will give you now,
to become firmly imprinted
into the automatic thinking part
of your mind,
the suggestion that
I give you now,
begin to affect you now,
and grow stronger
with each and every day,
Note: The Magical Forest Induction has concluded. Please insert the therapy suggestions from the end of this chapter.

Day at the Beach

it is a beautiful summer day,
you are walking with effortless ease
along a white sandy beach,
you feel the warmth of the sun
on your skin,
and the refreshing coolness
of the sea breeze as
it gently sprays against your skin,
you feel the white foam of
the rolling waves
as you watch those waves come
crashing into shore,
you feel peace and tranquility
rolling toward you,
you hear the sound of the waves,
as they gently crash upon the shore,
you hear the sound of the sea gulls,
as they gently rise and fall,
floating with effortless ease
on the salty sea breeze,
their wings extended,
as they float on a cushion of air,
you watch the graceful sea gulls
as they soar
higher and higher
into to the blue sky,
rising higher and higher,
then suddenly…
dropping…
down, down, down
to the aqua green waters of the ocean,
as you watch the seagulls in graceful flight,
you notice the sky is a dreamy blue,
and puffy white pillows of clouds
billow across that dreamy blue sky,
you can watch those clouds float

and drift,
your conscious mind
just begins to drift
as if drifting on a cloud,
drifting away for a time,
and the mind and the body,
just to began to relax with
and into
the comfortable white clouds,
and you can float and drift,
and dream away for a time,
and that is fine because
it all belongs to you,
in the distance you hear the sound
of children laughing,
the happy, blissful sound of laughter,
the sound is faint
yet distinguishable
if you listen very carefully
you may notice that your hearing
is becoming more and more acute,
you can feel the pleasant warmth
of the sand between your toes,
you can see the relaxing waves
rolling into the shore,
coming closer to you,
and you are drawn
to those waves,
as if drawn by a magnetic force,
an irresistible force,
drawing you
to it's peace and tranquility,
you are ten steps from the water,
as you walk toward the relaxing water,
your hand brushes against
your stomach,
and you notice
with a sense of pride,

how small your stomach really is
and as you look down
and survey your body,
you notice
the leanness, the firmness pf your body,
you can feel vitality energizing
every cell of your body,
you walk with your head held high,
with large portions of
self-confidence and self-assurance
apparent in every step you take,
you enjoy your health,
you enjoy the effortless way in which you move
you move with grace and agility,
feeling so proud of yourself
for allowing yourself to become
your ideal weight and size,
a smile begins to tug at the
corners of your mouth,
as you realize how easy it was
to allow the suggestions that
are receiving now,
to become
a permanent part of your
automatic thinking process,
these suggestions
have become a very powerful force
in enabling you
to create the body
you desire and deserve
now you are five steps from
the relaxing ocean waters,
those peaceful
and tranquil waters
just began to flow toward you,
and you notice,
the waves come in and out
in synchrony with your breathing,

as you breathe in
the waves come in,
coming closer to you,
as you breathe out
the waves go out,
moving away from you
for a time
each and every time
that you slowly inhale and exhale
in rhythm with the gently rocking waves
the waves come closer to you,
until you can feel
warm salty water just
licking over your feet,
leaving your feet
with a wonderful feeling of relaxation,
the waves come back
washing over your shins
and calves
leaving your shins
and calves
very loose, limp, and relaxed,
the ocean water washes
your knees,
lubricating your knees,
with a very warm, pleasant sensation
of relaxation,
the wave roll out to sea,
and all the stresses
and tensions of the day
just seem to disappear,
the waves wash
up to your thighs,
moving you gently
with a relaxing rocking motion,
as the waves go out to sea
all the minor and major muscle
aches and pains

just seem to disappear,
the water washes
to your stomach,
relaxing your stomach,
relaxing your fingers,
your hands, and
your lower back,
you can feel the tension
leaving your body,
the wave washes up to
your chest,
gently lifting you from the
ocean floor,
moving you
around with a very pleasant
rocking motion,
you become more
and more buoyant,
you become lighter and lighter,
until you realize,
that you are floating
gently, safely, and comfortably
in the arms
of the ocean
the ocean continues to gently rock you
in a soothing way,
the way a mother
would rock her child,
as you float,
in those tranquil,
gentle waters,
you can allow yourself
to become
more relaxed, more peaceful
more purposeful
than you have ever
known yourself to be,
and the mind and the body

just relax more and more
than before,
and the day passes in tranquility,
and soothing relaxation,
and as the sun just begins to set,
you look to the horizon
and see brilliant hues
of orange, yellow, purple, and gold
blazing across the horizon
reflecting their beauty in the
vast mirror of an endless ocean,
you find that you are relaxed
from the tips of your toes
to the top of your scalp,
the mind and the body
are most relaxed when
they relax together,
and you have known all along,
that it is so much easier to learn
when you are relaxed,
and now you are in a place
of peaceful relaxation,
a place of very powerful learning,
the suggestions which
I give to you now
begin to affect you now,
and become stronger
with each and every passing day,
Note: The Day at the Beach induction has concluded. Please insert the therapeutic suggestions listed at the close of this chapter.

Autumn in the Mountains

It is a beautiful, brisk, autumn day
in the mountains,
you enjoy breathing
the clean mountain air,
you breathe
in deep, relaxing, breaths,
you are high in the mountains,
and you can see for miles
below you,
down the mountainside,
down to the lowlands,
down to the pastures,
you are amazed
at the panorama
of vivid colors you see before you,
fall is in the crisp air,
and you see
the autumn leaves falling down,
falling in brilliant hues of
gold, yellow, orange, red,
silver, gray, white, brown,
platinum, black, and white
you see these colors
and a countless number of nameless shades,
breathtaking colors
in all the subtle shades
in the color spectrum,
you may find yourself wondering
how many variations of colors
that there really are,
how many variations of colors
for the color green
or the color blue,
as you wonder about those colors
you find your mind wandering
as you wander

up a mountain trail
that twists, turns
and gradually winds
it's way to the mountain top,
working its way up the great mountain,
a mountain so tall that
the top of the top is lost
to your eyes
in a cloud like mist
as you move
with grace, agility, and effortless ease,
you can find your conscious
mind
wondering
if this is the way Jack felt,
when he climbed up the beanstalk,
energy flows to you
from the trees,
you feel energy, vitality, and bliss
coursing through your body,
as your lean, fit, powerful body
carries you up
this winding mountain trail,
you can hear the pleasant crunching sounds
of leaves beneath
your hiking boots,
you can feel the soft, comforting feel
of the pillow like leaves beneath your feet,
as you walk with
powerful, gliding strides
which easily move you
up this grand mountain,
you can smell the
scents around you,
scents of pine, juniper
and rich fertile earth,
these smells only
heighten the sense of tranquility

and peacefulness
that you are experiencing,
all your senses
seem to be heightened
your awareness is amazing,
you even notice the
slight movement
of a squirrel
in a beautiful tree
just below you,
while just above you,
the sound of the birds
seems to be blended into
one marvelous and relaxing song,
as your conscious mind
just begins to drift off
in relaxation,
while your unconscious mind,
begins to write
the lyrics
to the music
of the mountains,
you feel the quiet, comfortable harmony
of nature,
you can feel the power of the mountains,
the mountains are
strong, enduring and nurturing,
the mountains surround
and protect you
as a mother would protect her child,
and you relax with every sound you hear,
even the sound of your own breathing,
even the sound of your own heart,
as the healthy beat of your heart,
becomes a soothing sound,
in the background of your mind,
and you can drift away for a time
as your body climbs

and your spirit soars,
your body feels light and
you climb with effortless ease
up this magnificent mountain,
you power up this mountain
because you are fit and healthy,
and it feels so good
to have so much energy
to accomplish
so many things
and you smile with a profound
sense of gratitude,
because it feels so good
to be your ideal weight and size,
and it feels so good
for you to know
that you have allowed your body
to become its perfect weight and size,
by allowing the suggestions
that I give to you now
to become
a permanent part
of your
automatic thinking
become as automatic as
your breathing,
as you breath in relaxation,
as you breathe out tension
and stress,
your breathing and your climbing
become synchronized,
as you climb,
you inhale relaxation
with every breath,
and as you exhale
you breathe out stress and tension
with each and every breath,
and the mind and the body

just begin to relax
more and more
than before,
relaxing more deeply,
relaxing more and more completely
with each and every breath,
until it almost seems as if
you are floating up the mountain,
almost as if
you were striding on air,
and you may begin to wonder
if you are striding on air
or on a cushion of soft
and colorful autumn leaves,
until it just seems to take
too much effort to try to take
the effort it takes to
even bother to
tell the difference
knowing that the difference
really makes no difference,
to the relaxation which
you are experiencing,
it is so much easier,
to simply allow your mind
to dream and drift and drop
just dropping down
as a falling leaf drops from
that beautiful mountain top
just dropping down from
the highlands
to the lowlands
just allowing your mind
to float on that leaf,
with that leaf,
floating down into the valley
of peaceful relaxation and tranquility,
as your mind drifts down

your body climbs up,
until you reach the peak
of this magnificent, misty, and majestic mountain,
when you are at the peak
of the mountain top,
you will be at the peak
of your suggestibility,
and you will enter
a very serene and peaceful log cabin
known as deep, deep, hypnosis,
you are standing in a comfortable cloud
on top of the mountain,
you are walking comfortably
and safely through this cloud,
then a strong wind blows
and simply whisks the cloud away
leaving you smiling
as you look
at a very peaceful
and comfortable
log cabin
you can see the white puffs of smoke
as they billow up from
a friendly fireplace,
as the smoke billows up,
you can see it linger for awhile
against the blue sky
and then it is gone
simply merging with
and disappearing into
that dreamy blue sky,
you begin to feel the chill
of the mountain air
as night comes quickly
in the mountains,
you place your hand
in your pocket
for warmth,

and in that pocket,
you discover a key,
you find within in your own pocket
a key that fits,
a key that fits the cabin door,
you realize with a sense of amusement
that this is your cabin,
this cabin high above the city
high above all the stresses and tensions
of the day
belongs to you,
the cabin seems to be
welcoming you home,
you use the key
and enter this
strangely familiar cabin,
as you do
you see the inviting blaze
of a friendly fire
in the fireplace,
you feel the relaxing warmth
of the fireplace,
you see an inviting rug and
many soft pillows,
you lie on the rug
and make yourself
more comfortable
than you have ever been before,
and as you do
you begin to feel the
relaxing warmth
of the fireplace,
you begin to feel that warmth
beckoning to you,
and that warmth
just begins to relax
each and every toe
on your feet,

as that relaxing warmth
begins to spread to your feet,
begins to seep into
your ankles,
flowing into your calves
and shins,
relaxing and lubricating
your knees
with a pleasant warm feeling
and that feeling
of relaxation
which spreads
to your upper legs,
relaxing your inner thighs,
relaxing your outer thighs,
and you can experience that warmth
occurring in your lap,
and as it does
it quickly spreads
to your hips,
relaxing your hips,
curving to your stomach,
as it does
you can feel
that wonderful sensation spreading
to your lower back,
just relaxing all the muscles
of the lower back,
then this wonderful sensation of relaxation
finds the spinal column,
and slowly begins
to climb the up the spinal column,
relaxing each and every vertebra
on the way up,
and spreading relaxation in both directions,
relaxing and warming
all the muscles
of the upper back

and shoulders,
just curving around to your chest,
relaxing the chest with radiant warmth,
now your stomach is relaxed,
and your chest is relaxed,
and all the internal organs inside
just seem to slow down
with relaxation and warmth,
and you can feel the warmth
in your neck
in your neck
all the stresses and tensions
of the day
just want to accumulate,
but as that warm feeling flows
into your neck,
you can feel all the stresses and tensions
of the day being chased away,
you can feel the warmth on your face,
on your ears, and your scalp,
and now you are relaxed
from the
top of your head
to the tips of your toes,
as your body relaxes
your mind relaxes as well,
relaxes with it
into it
because you have known
all along
that you can learn more easily
when you are relaxed,
and now you have entered
into a very powerful place
of relaxation and learning,
a very wonderful, peaceful place
known as deep, deep hypnosis,
and in this state of perfect relaxation and learning

you will accept the suggestions
you are receiving,
the suggestions are accepted
into a very deep
and powerful place
in the unconscious mind,
and these suggestions
will begin to effect you now
and will become stronger
each and every passing day,
Note: The Autumn in the Mountains induction has concluded. Please insert the
therapeutic suggestions listed at the conclusion of this chapter.

Luxury Hotel

it is a beautiful spring day,
as you step out of your house,
you see a very elegant
long white limousine,
the limousine gracefully enters into
your driveway,
you are wearing your favorite clothes,
and they fit so very perfectly,
you feel so comfortable and attractive,
in these new clothes,
and you notice
the admiring glances of
your neighbors and friends
as they watch the chauffeur
open the limousine door for you,
you slide inside
moving with grace and elegance,
moving lightly and easily
almost as if
you are floating,
you sit back of the beautiful car,
the comfortable, plush leather seats
of the fine automobile
impart a wonderful feeling
of relaxation,
you listen to your favorite music.
and you enjoy the words
and the music,
as you enjoy the ride
the temperature in the limousine
is absolutely perfect
and the ride is as smooth as
floating on a magic carpet
you find yourself
beginning to drift off
with relaxation,

just drifting off
and drifting back
to the surface
of wakeful awareness
at times,
and it feels so good
to allow
someone else to drive
for a time
and it feels so good,
to allow
someone else
to handle
all the details
for a time,
time flies
you arrive
at your five-star luxury hotel,
your suite has already been
paid for
and someone has taken care of all the details,
the bell boy
carries your luggage,
and shows you to your penthouse suite,
you walk crisply and lightly through
the opulent and tastefully decorated lobby,
you notice the smiles
and the admiring glances
from the numerous
guests at this elegant hotel,
and it feels so good to know
that you have become
your perfect weight and size,
it feels so good to know
that you have become
firm, fit, attractive, and sexy
simply by allowing the suggestions
that you receive

to deeply sink
into the automatic thinking
center of your unconscious mind,
all the guests are well dressed and
very well mannered,
you receive many compliments
about your physical appearance,
many guests remark
that you are a very attractive person,
you enjoy the attention,
which you are receiving,
you follow the bell boy
to the elevator
and you notice
the beautiful and peaceful lobby area,
you can fee this is a place
of perfect relaxation and pleasure,
as you enter into the stylish glass elevator,
you have a sense of contentment,
the elevator ascends very comfortably and very safely,
you enjoy the ride,
your spirits rise higher and higher
as the glass elevator ascends
higher and higher,
the panoramic view below is
quite spectacular,
the hotel is quiet, peaceful
and very relaxing,
the bell boy opens the door
to your room
and you see
the most amazing and magnificent
hotel room that you could ever
possibly imagine,
you are drawn to a very beautiful hot tub
you watch the warm water in the hot tub
swirl and as if by magic
you discover yourself

relaxing in this wonderful hot tub,
you can feel the relaxing warmth
spreading through your toes
flowing through your feet
swirling around your calves and shins
relaxing your knees,
this wonderful sensation of relaxation
begins to flow into your legs
your inner thighs relax,
your outer thighs relax,
as the water swirls
around your lap and hips,
you can enjoy a pleasant, warm
and relaxing feeling
as it grows and flows
to your waist
to your lower back
and to your spinal column
where all the connections
of the body
just seem to be,
and all the connections
to the body
just begin to experience
a feeling
of profound relaxation,
one vertebra at a time,
and the relaxation
flows to the top of the spinal column
spreading out to relax all the major
and all the minor muscles
of the upper back,
as it does
it just begins to swirl around
to the chest
and now the chest, back, and stomach
are relaxed,
and all the internal organs inside

just seem to relax as well,
and as the internal organs slow down
in relaxation,
you can feel the relaxation flowing
through your shoulders,
into your neck,
all the tensions and stresses
of the day
just seem to want to go to
and to accumulate in the neck,
but this wonderfully, warm water
from the relaxing hot-tub
just touches the neck
and all the tensions and stresses
of the day
just seem to disappear,
the face relaxes,
the area between
the mouth and ears
may become
so relaxed
that the mouth
may have a tendency
to just want to
part ever so slightly
in relaxation
and if it does
that it is fine
because it all belongs to you,
and now you are relaxed
from the tips of your toes
to the top of your scalp,
you find yourself comfortable
and refreshed
as you step out of the hot-tub
and prepare to meet good friends
in the lobby of the hotel,
with effortless ease

you become ready,
when you see yourself
in the golden mirror,
you find with a sense of amazement, amusement
and pride that you
are so very attractive,
you leave your room
wearing the absolute
perfect clothes for you,
you feel so slender, comfortable
and attractive in your new clothes,
as you step inside the elegant and safe
glass elevator,
you can see the lobby through the glass,
the lobby is the most beautiful,
relaxing and peaceful lobby that
you could ever possibly imagine,
you push the down button,
and as you do you,
feel the elevator safely
and smoothly begin to descend,
you feel yourself going deeper
and deeper into a place of
wonderful relaxation,
a place of complete profound peacefulness,
a place called deep, deep hypnosis,
you notice that you are now on floor ten
of the elegant hotel,
as you count down the floors,
you begin to go down, down,
you know that when you reach the count
of zero,
you will have reached the peak of
your suggestibility,
and when you reach the count of zero,
you will be in a place of deep relaxation
and very powerful learning,
known as deep, deep hypnosis,

you find yourself self counting down now,
ten…nine…letting go and
going deeper…eight…seven…
just experiencing a wonderful feeling of
letting go and relaxation,
relaxing more and more than before
six…five…going deeper…and even deeper,
four…deeper and deeper than before…
going down quickly now…three…two…
one…DEEP SLEEP…
now you are in a very powerful
place of learning,
you are free to accept the following suggestions
into the automatic thinking center
of your unconscious mind,
Note: The Luxury Hotel progressive relaxation has concluded. Simply give the
suggestions listed on the next page.

Suggestions:

In the past I have identified with
eating the wrong
kinds of food
and with being overweight,
I now will change my patterns
of thinking and eating so
that I will become thinner,
before I began to eat a meal,
I take a very deep breath,
releasing the air very slowly,
and as I remember to breathe deeply
I remember to eat my food more slowly,
I take deep cleansing breaths
this deep breathing
serves as a reminder to me
to eat my food more slowly,
I begin to find
that I eat my food
more and more slowly,
savoring each and every bite,
I know the true pleasure of eating
comes from the taste,
the texture, and the aroma
of the food,
and I know that the
taste, texture, and aroma
of food
can be enjoyed more and more
simply by eating more slowly
than before,
That's right,
I find that I begin to eat
my food more slowly
savoring each and every bite
enjoying the taste of food more as
I eat more slowly,

I enjoy eating smaller bites
chewing and swallowing
my food before
I take another bite,
I discover I am happiest
whenever I eat my food
at a more relaxed pace
and when I do
my food tastes more
delicious,
by eating slowly
I allow my unconscious mind
enough time
to send to me a signal,
when I receive this signal
I know that I have eaten
just the right amount of food
for me,
just the right amount of food
to satisfy the nutritional needs
of my body,
I find when I receive this signal
I am completely satisfied,
comfortable, and happy,
I find myself pushing my plate
a few inches from me,
and as I push my plate from me
I lose all wish to eat further,
knowing that if I try to past
the point of perfect nutritional comfort
and satisfaction,
I will discover
each bite past
the point of nutritional comfort
will only lead to
discomfort,
a bloated feeling,
a feeling of lethargy,

in order to avoid these
painful consequences of
overeating
I simply stop eating
when I have reached the place
of perfect nutritional comfort and satisfaction,
I know when my body is full
and I am happy and content
to quit eating when I am full and
satisfied,
I enjoy leaving food on my plate
because I know that I really
don't need all that food and
I really don't want it,
each and every day
I find that I am more drawn to foods
that are high in protein and
low in carbohydrates,
those foods that promote lean muscle
taste better with each passing day,
I find I lose the taste for foods
that promote the accumulation of
massive amounts of fatty tissue,
I enjoy eating high protein foods,
I can feel my body becoming leaner
and more toned,
if I *try* to eat foods that are wrong for me
I discover that after a bite or two
these foods leave a very unpleasant taste
in my mouth,
coating my tongue with a
very nasty and disgusting taste,
but I know I can quickly
cleanse my pallet
of this nasty taste
by drinking a glass or bottle
of delicious water,
whenever I have the passing thought

of eating something fattening
I am reminded that
nothing tastes as good as thin feels,
whenever I notice that I have a wish
to eat something that is bad for me,
I also notice that I have a
strong burning desire to
enjoy feeling,
the power of refusing to eat
unhealthy and fattening food,
I will remember that
nothing tastes as good
as thin feels,
if I still have a wish to
try to eat fattening food,
I will not deny that small wish
but I will taste the
fattening food
one small bite at a time,
placing a small bite of food on
the very tip of my tongue
where my sense of taste is
most acute,
when I chew that small bite
very carefully
I think about what I am eating
and my sense of taste becomes heightened,
I begin to taste
all the processed sugar,
all the preservatives,
all the chemical additives,
that are packed into that
unhealthy food,
as I chew that unhealthy food slowly and
taste all the ingredients
that are
essentially poisonous to my
health, happiness, and physical appearance

I begin to notice
this type of food leaves a
very nasty taste in my mouth,
I will find myself losing
all desire to eat
more than a bite or two,
I find that I
quickly and easily cleanse
my pallet
of this nasty taste by
drinking a glass
or bottle of water,
water is becoming
my beverage of choice
at meal time and
in between meals as well,
frequently I have a very powerful
thirst for water,
frequently my lips become
very dry and parched
my tongue becomes
very thick and
my throat becomes
very dry and parched,
and I find myself thinking
about drinking
delicious water,
if I try to drink any other
beverage, I discover that
drinking this other beverage only
increases the dry thirsty feeling that
I am experiencing,
the more I try to drink
a beverage other than
water
the thirstier that
I become.
I know that in order to

truly quench and satisfy
my great thirst,
I must drink delicious water,
I feel good about drinking
water because I know that
drinking water will energize
and cleanse my body,
drinking water will
give my metabolism a boost
and it will accelerate my weight loss,
I know that drinking water is
one of the healthiest habits
that I can develop,
I know that these suggestions become
stronger and stronger
each day and every day,
and more and more automatic
each and every day,
I know that drinking water is
as important as breathing air,
and it is becoming as automatic,
I begin to feel a very pleasant
warming sensation
coursing through my body,
I know that my metabolism
is becoming heightened,
I can feel the warmth caressing
and coursing
through my skin,
I can feel this pleasant sensation spreading
through my arms and legs,
I can experience the pleasure
of this relaxing sensation,
and the joy of having so much energy
to accomplish so many things,
as my metabolism burns
hotter and hotter,
I experience a surge of energy

and a surge of motivation
enabling me to enjoy
moving my body briskly
while doing my favorite exercise,
as my body pleasantly and comfortably
becomes warmer and warmer,
I imagine my extra pounds
simply melting away,
melting away with effortless ease,
I can concentrate on raising my metabolism
and feeling this wonderful warmth
at any time at all,
because it all belongs to me
I enjoy this mental exercise,
and I enjoy accelerating my weight loss
more and more
each and every day,
as I follow my weight loss program,
I begin to discover that
I enjoy exercising my body,
it feels so good to move
my body rhythmically
as I walk, run, dance, swim, or exercise,
I enjoy increasing the warmth of my body
until I can feel a very pleasant glistening
of perspiration caressing my skin,
it feels good to know that
I am elevating my metabolism
and that I will benefit from
the after-burn of calories
long after I am through exercising,
each and every step I take,
each and every movement or
repetition that I make,
brings me closer to my goal,
I know with each movement
of my body
I am becoming

leaner, fitter, healthier, and more attractive,
each and every time that I exercise
it becomes easier and easier
because my physical condition improves
each and every time that I exercise,
when I exercise it feels as if I enter
into a zone of time distortion,
and twenty minutes of exercise
begins to feel like only ten,
as I move my body continually for a few minutes
I discover my second wind,
and then I know that I can exercise
tirelessly for extended periods of time,
I find myself wanting to eat my largest meal
at noon when the sun is at the highest point
in the sky,
I am so nutritionally satisfied
from my noon meal
that I find
I have a growing desire
to eat smaller meals in the evening,
I find that I lose desire
to eat past seven o'clock at night,
and because I don't eat past seven o'clock
I find that I sleep
more quickly and comfortably
throughout the night,
when my head touches the pillow
I begin to drift
into a very peaceful slumber,
sleeping quickly, deeply, and soundly
throughout the night,
dreaming a wonderful dream and
awakening in the morning
refreshed, energized, invigorated, and
highly motivated to follow my
weight loss program,
these suggestions begin to

affect me now and become
stronger and stronger
with each and every passing day,
Note: Listen to these as you go to sleep at night and allow yourself to drift into a
peaceful sleep.

23

The Become Thin and Stay Thin Recipe

I want to congratulate you for reading up to this point. I know that your desire to become thin is strong. Your faith will grow as you use the techniques that you have learned. I know that when you apply the principles presented here to your life you will mentally create your ideal weight.

I promised you a recipe to become thin and stay thin. Here it is. The main ingredients are desire, faith, imagination, and persistence. Begin with large portions of desire, mix well with your imagination, heat that imaginative desire until it is boiling hot; add faith and persistence, and stir until the mixture has become a habit.

I would like to leave you with some poetic, uplifting, or profound words, but the truth is the fundamentals of weight loss are simply desire, faith, imagination, and persistence. In this book, you have been given many techniques to help you develop your desire, faith, imagination, and persistence. With the use of these four qualities, your weight loss is assured.

Throughout this book I have tried to be very focused on practical techniques for weight loss. I have to tell you that I feel a very strong kinship with you. Without knowing you individually, I know a lot about you. I know that you are among the small percentage of people who are willing to open their hearts and minds to new ideas. You are a person who is willing to accept responsibility for the conditions of your life, and to take positive action to change those conditions. You have the ability to dream and to imagine. You have the courage, intelligence, and determination to explore new ways of thinking. You are willing to invest the time it takes to improve yourself. You have my respect and admiration, and I wish you well.

I know that when you apply and master the principles that you have learned here, you will lose all the weight that you desire. You will be healthier, happier, fitter, and more attractive. I want you to know that not only will your body have transformed, but your character will have transformed as well. By looking at, weighing, and measuring your body, you will have discovered that these principles really work. *You will be the proof that these techniques work.* You will end your struggle with weight for life, but you will have only begun to tap the surface of what these principles can do for you.

I know that you are so much more than your physical body, and no matter how incredible your physique or figure becomes, it can never match you inner beauty. Once you have learned to control your mind in one area, you will have the faith required to know that you can control your life in other areas such as relationships, finances, and your relationship with God (in whatever manner it manifests itself). My fervent wish for you is that your life be filled with health, happiness, and a great abundance of love.

Note to the reader

If you ever discover that you are not moving in the direction of your weight loss goal, a simple analysis will reveal that you have had a breakdown in either intensity of desire, your faith, or the persistence of your efforts. At this point, you can simply use hypnosis, the Power of Pretend, the Power of Questions, the Law of Reverse Suggestion, the Law of Dominant Suggestion, and the Power of Emotions to get back on track.

Consider this: all elite athletes need a coach. A coach can add perspective; a coach can encourage and give insight that inspires you to achieve your goals. If you are dead serious about losing weight, then I would like to be your *personal coach*. You can call or email me to find out more about my hypnosis and coaching sessions.

I will be conducting seminars and doing book signings and individual sessions in your area. If you are interested in attending a seminar, book singing, or scheduling a session, please contact me by email at **lancemo@sbcglobal.net** or call me at **432-684-5221.**

Here is a priced list of products

Hypnosis Weight Loss CD...$19.95 (add $4.50 for shipping & handling)

Audio Seminar... $49.95 (add $5.00 for shipping and handling)

$5.00 off the purchase of any Hypnosis Weight Loss Center Product

---

$20.00 off the Price of a Hypnosis Session at the Hypnosis Weight Loss Center

0-595-30405-2

www.ingramcontent.com/pod-product-compliance
Lightning Source LLC
Chambersburg PA
CBHW061305280526
45784CB00002B/908